MW01264223

The Gospel According To Chubby

By Jeremy Rochford

The Gospel According to Chubby by Jeremy Rochford
ISBN: 978-0-9843223-0-5

For correspondence:
Jeremy@JeremyRochford.com

Jeremy Rochford
Po Box 128076
Nashville TN, 37212

JeremyRochford.com

Cover design by Media Series
Photography by Joe Ortiz
Copyright 2009, 2010 by Jeremy Rochford
All Rights Reserved

Table of Contents

Foreword

There I was, minding my own business. Sitting backstage reading through my notes getting ready to preach to a packed auditorium and I looked across the room and saw one of the musicians...well...uh....he was kind of rubbing his chest...in a weird way. It caught me off guard and he looked up and I was busted. I had a puzzled look on my face and it just popped out, "What are you doing?!" He said that he was fixing his shirt so it wouldn't get caught on his "moobs". Okay, I'm pretty hip-to-the-lingo-yo but I didn't have a clue what he was talking about. He explained that the "moob" was a gathering of chub on the chest of overweight men. Oh, Moob. I get it. I was looking at him and thought he was just cracking a joke and kicked back, "You're not overweight." That's when he dropped the bomb, "Yeah, I have lost 200lbs."

I sat there unimpressed until he whipped out a "before" pic. Holy Moley! He did drop a ton...or at least 10% of a ton! I was a little more impressed but not much. I became overly impressed and a huge (heh, get it?) fan when he told me about his journey. Everything from food addiction to the little things that continued to spiral him out of control. Jeremy told me about the ridicule that happened overtly and the ridicule that happened in his own mind. And the thing that blew me away is that he didn't have any surgery, no lipo, no lapband, he did it the old fashion way...he focused himself. What made him do what he did, think the way he thought, feel the way he felt. As we parted I was officially blown away.

This book will tell you about his journey. Whatever your issue, compulsion or hang-up is you will see yourself in the pages. My issue has never been food, but I can relate to where he has been and what he has gone through and I find encouragement for my own failings.

Warning: This is not a politically correct book. There will be a lot of people who will get all offended about the way he writes. "Oh, you shouldn't say that kind of stuff." "People can't help it." "Don't say that about yourself." For those people, buy this book and pass it on. It's not for you.

Jeremy does not sensationalize his story. But he doesn't candy coat it either. He will lay out everything about his physical, emotional, and social decay and will let you know that the biggest issue was his spiritual decay. He doesn't allow anyone to sit back and say, "Oh, I have a thyroid issue," or "I'm just chunky." He calls it like he sees it. Not by pointing the finger saying, "Look at you." He does it by raising his hand saying, "Look at me. I have a problem. And I found the answer."

The Gospel According to Chubby is not the end. This is only the beginning of the story. It is a remarkable journey of one of the more that 150 million overweight Americans who are searching to fill an emptiness of their soul with food. It is one persons journey of victory and defeat, fears and hopes. And it is one persons journey from stealing to buy food to becoming a certified personal trainer. That's right, from being the fatty to being the fat-loss coach!

You are not alone on your journey. I know it's difficult. It's frustrating and nothing seems to work. I know this is a cliché, but I know Jeremy and it is so true, "If he can do it, so can you!"

-Justin Lookadoo
International Speaker
Best Selling Author of *Dateable: are you? are they?*
www.lookadoo.com

Prologue

Oh you have got to be kidding me,
this can't be happening now!
Why is this happening now?

> You know, if you just stop squirming
> maybe we can wiggle it in.

I understand that.
I'm squirming because every time you push
down you're pinching a stomach roll.

> Sir, this is no time for joking.
> If we can't get this to lock, we can't let you ride.
> I have been trying for the past 15 minutes,
> so now is not the time to be funny.

I'm not trying to be funny,
you are physically hurting me!
Every time you push down you pinch
my skin and the harder you push,
the harder it is to breathe.

> I'm sorry sir; there just is no other way.
> Every time I get close, my fingers slip
> from your sweat. Can you sweat less?

Are you serious? I'm uncomfortable as it is
and now people are gathering around because
of the scene were making.

I just don't know what I can do.
Hold on, let me get my boss.
"HEY RICHIE, CAN YOU COME HERE?"

Fantastic!?!

Yeah? What's the problem?

Well, this gentleman would like to ride the go-karts,
however, we can't seem to get him to fit.

We'll that's not a problem.
We can seat him in the #22 car.
That car is reserved for our "huskier" guests.

Um...

What is it?

This is the #22 car.

Are you sure?

Yup.

Oh. Hmm… Well…

Is there some sort of extender we can use?

Um. Not really. No. Well, yes. But. Um.

For safety reasons they're already built into the #22 car. Because of our insurance, we equipped at least one car with a harness system built for a...well...um...more "manly" man.

Sir? Are you okay?

You look like you're crying.

Oh me? Ha ha...no...it's just the sun.
Sunscreen, you know...the sweat...
in my eyes...heat...yeah. The sun.
I'm fine.

Are you sure?

Yeah, (tear) fine.

*Here. What if we
just pull this like this...*

OH SNAPPP! COME ON!
OH MAN THAT HURTS!!!

*Well if you would
just stop squirming…*

I'M SQUIRMING BECAUSE
YOU ARE HURTING ME!!!

3

Sir, stop yelling!
You are the one who got us into this.
Well, actually you are the one who is
preventing us from getting you into this.

What?

Nothing.
It's just in all of my years of running this ride,
I have never seen this happen. Ever.
I just don't know what else to do.

So, what are you saying?

What I am saying is that in every summer I have
come to this boardwalk as a patron,
as a ride operator, and now as a manager ,
I have never seen anyone turned away from this ride
because they could not fit. Now I have to do just that.
Sir we have tried everything, and you are
not fitting into the safety harness. I'm sorry sir,
you are going to have to leave. Now, would you
please step this way as to not further hold up the line.

What!?! Are you serious!?!

Sir, I am really sorry.
But I have a line and you do not fit safely in the car.
I am very sorry, but I am going to have to ask you to leave.

Chapter 1:

In the Beginning

Have you ever wondered what a day in the life of a superstar is like? Forget the fame and the money, I wonder how it feels to wake up and be that perfect hybrid of attribute and ability. It seems these days that, more times than not, ice hockey players are able to ice skate before they're able to walk. Basketball players are able to dribble on the court before they're accidentally dribbling on themselves. Musicians are emerging who can harmonize before they have the ability to speak. Even NASCAR drivers are winning track championships before they hit puberty, let alone are old enough to qualify for a driver's license.

But what about the other half? Those of us who are born with the very same characteristics, but instead of having the desire to change the world, we have the desire for a value meal? Let me tell you my story. My infatuation with eating began a mere eight minutes after I was born. Four hundred eighty seconds after I took my first breath, my mother was taken out of recovery to feed her brand new baby boy. (Skating since you were two, Gretzky? Amateur!) Admittedly, one of the saving graces about early childhood is that everyone is little chubby. And, for a little while, it's adorable.

"Aw, look at little Jeremy getting into that ice cream.
He has such a healthy appetite!"

That's what you always say to little fat kids, right?

"You have a healthy appetite.
You are going to grow up big and strong, aren't you?"

But what if that kid grows into an adult where "big" and "strong" are not intertwined? No one ever seems to intervene with...

"Oh my gosh, that kid looks like a van! Doesn't he realize
that his social life will be miserable and his self esteem will
be non-existent? Someone should stop him now!"

But that is grown-up talk. Kids don't worry about social lives. All kids worry about are cookies, cakes, and that fantastic penny candy store two blocks from the house. Two blocks, indeed. One of my fondest childhood memories occurred in first grade: the day my sister introduced me to Abers. Abers was a quaint little candy store located parallel to the elementary school I attended. To me, it was heaven. Instead of streets of gold, I saw rows of sugar. This is how heaven was dispensed:

> 1 Cent Tier - All the gummy candies one could think of. Norwegish Fish, Sour Apples, Sour Watermelons, Sour Peaches, Sour Field Kids, and Gummi Bears. There were so many and I loved them all.

> 5 Cent Tier - This row was clearly for the upperclassmen. It included Gummi Peach Rings, Big Norwegish Fish, and those little flying saucer things with tiny sprinkles in them. I don't know what they are

formally called, but they tasted like a communion wafer with miniature candy pellets inside. This was the altar at which I worshipped. Unfortunately, I was too young to have a job, so my funding was limited. It was my lack of funding that stifled my appreciation for this tier.

10 Cent Tier - I liked to call this the special occasion tier. In fact, the only time I could even consider this prestigious row was when holiday money came into play. Cows Tales, Sixlet Miniatures, and individually wrapped licorice anchored this tier. This was a great row, but at the age of six, money was scarce. I had to choose my pleasures wisely. I was a quantity over quality kind of lad, so I championed the penny rack for as long as I could.

Oh Abers, such a beautiful romance. Who could tamper with such a pure and adoring love? The Pennsylvania State Board of Education, that's who! As it turns out, the statistical data from my first grade physical confirmed something my parents were already beginning to think. My "kids' meal"-sized weight issue was quickly becoming a "super-sized" adult problem. My permanent record speaks for itself.

"Six-year old male, mildly obese. This is due in part to snacking. Parents also aware. Dieting since February, three meals, afternoon fruit snack, NO CANDY... Some teasing at school seems to tolerate well. Advise nutritional awareness."

Let me break this down for you. I was six years old, and I was on a diet. But also, let me put this into perspective, I was on a 1987 diet. The vintage food pyramid suggested that I snag one item per food group, per meal. Technically, this could be achieved through a serving of Hamburger Assistor with a side of

Hungry Bob boxed mashed potatoes, all of which were staples in the Rochford pantry. You might notice the statement above that reads, "Parents also aware." That statement refers more to their awareness of the overweight situation; it doesn't really allude to their awareness of what might be *causing* the situation.

In terms of the "No Candy" statement, well, let's just say that everything I mentioned during that physical might not have been entirely accurate. I worked hard to keep my Abers activity away from their knowing eyes. Let's be logical for a moment. Does a six-year-old child really gain enough excess weight to be diet-worthy on three meals a day and one afternoon snack of fruit?

I was obviously sneaking food from somewhere. Now that I knew they were watching me, I decided to make a game out of it. First I restricted my eating to all the places my parents were not. Walks home with diversions into the woods and back alleys became commonplace. I admit, this was not the safest option for a six-year-old; but with the control my parents had within the walls of our household, my options were limited.

My parents had no idea why I kept gaining weight. They felt my eating regiment was controlled. They thought what I ate was healthy. But they were oblivious to the other influences surrounding me. They concluded my continuing weight gain was due to the absence of exercise. Clearly if the boy is eating structured meals and still gaining weight, then it's his activity level that needs modification.

What could possibly be the greatest cure for inactivity in a six-year-old boy? Why, youth soccer, of course! What is there not to like about soccer? I mean, as a socially awkward, Easter-egg-looking six-year-old with the coordination of a log, why wouldn't I like the idea of running up and down a 100-yard field for an hour or so? Good times! This is where my finely honed talent of deliberately falling down finally found its purpose. I used it to comply with my parent's desire for my soccer involvement, yet I was able to avoid actually running. Genius, I know. By using this ability, I was able to secure the starting goaltender position for the entire season, completely nullifying whatever positive affects their plan might have had.

As an added bonus, there was a treat structure to every game. Who knew? The system was designed to reward victory. If we won the game, we were rewarded with a giant Little Deborah snack cake. To keep from hurting anyone's feelings, even our losing efforts earned a consolation Little Deborah. It was much smaller than the "snack cake of victory", but at least it was something. The possibility of a giant snack cake only made me work that much harder. And, the more I could eat in public, the less I had to sneak around. This winning philosophy helped me gain 15 pounds that spring and summer. As you can see, my parents' soccer intervention did not go as planned.

Halfway through the next season, my parents invested in the spoils of cable television. This may seem irrelevant now, but it was a turning point in my life Before you go ahead and make assumptions, I know what you're thinking: with cable TV, I strapped myself to a couch for hours on end, all the while eating myself to death, right? Come on gang, I can't go out like that. It was actually quite the opposite. Cable television would prove to be inspirational. It gave me a dream. It made me want to play professional baseball. Baseball? What? Allow me to explain. Somehow, through the graces of God, our suburban Pittsburgh cable package included the flagship networks from the New

York, Atlanta, and Chicago metropolitan areas. This meant that every night I had the choice of watching the Pittsburgh Pirates, the Chicago Cubs, the Atlanta Braves, or the New York Mets. It never got old; there was a different game every night!

It was a great time to become a baseball fan. The Mets had Dwight Gooden and Darryl Strawberry. The Cubs had Ryne Sandberg, Mark Grace, and some rookie named Greg Maddox. The Braves were winning everything, and last but not least, my hometown Pirates. This was the closest my generation would come to having a reason to cheer for black and gold baseball. With players like Barry Bonds, Bobby Bonilla, and Andy Van Slyke, those were good times.

So what was it about baseball that grabbed my attention? Was it the 95 mile-per-hour fastball? Was it the sound of the bat as it forced another baseball away from its home? Was it the smell of the field on opening day? Heck no! It was the fact that the players spent half of the game sitting on the bench eating. I mean, people got paid millions for this! Sunflower seeds, bubble gum, and the occasional chew (which I thought was beef jerky) were all on the game day menu.

Now, if there is one thing I learned from my year of sporting success, it was this: sports offer not only a chance for friendship, but also a public forum in which even mediocre and poor efforts are rewarded. Sometimes, those "Congratulations, you didn't win but at least you showed up!" awards were in the form of medallions. In my case, they were snacks. Since my parents monitored my food intake to insure I was eating "healthy" by their standards, I had to score as much good stuff as I could away from the house. Baseball seemed like the perfect opportunity to do just that. Victorious pizza parties and "you tried your best" snow cones were a fantastic fringe benefit of participation. I thrived on the fact that my mother couldn't stop me from eating when she was all the way in the bleachers and I was in the dugout. Baseball was no longer reserved for champions. It was now a place for me!

It didn't take too much effort to convince my parents that baseball was the best exercise option, because I had already convinced them I was on their side for this weight loss effort. When the next spring's Little League registration rolled around, we were first in line. However, my birth date made me ineligible to play that year. This meant that I could either sit out an entire year while I waited for Little League eligibility, or I could play a season of tee ball. That was not cool. I was already larger than most kids my age, now I had the honor of eclipsing a team filled with kids two to three years younger than me. However, knowing that tee ball allowed me to leave the house and eat food that wasn't a part of my weight loss regimen was all the convincing I needed.

I wore a fake smile that proved very useful, as my first attempt at tee ball would be nothing short of a comedy of errors, figuratively and literally. Clearly I was a liability when it came to running, but I had no idea I wasn't able to catch or hit the ball. I figured my 2-3 years of added maturity, as well as my athletic prowess from goaltending would allow me to rise quickly through the ranks and take the team by storm.

Wow, was I wrong. I was so bad at tee ball that I they assigned me the role of catcher. Now, let me be clear. In 95% of baseball plays, the catcher is an integral part of the team. They communicate with the pitcher concerning pitch selection, they calm the players down in high pressure situations, they are like a field general. In real baseball, it is an honor to be a catcher. In tee ball, not so much. You see, in tee ball, a catcher is nothing more than a target that chases the ball around the batter's box after it hits him in the stomach. I was getting purple nurples in the form of baseball contusions. It was embarrassing. My inability to crouch down didn't help matters. I was too much of a Weeble to keep my balance. Did I mention our uniforms were orange? They were. So instead of being called "The Great Pumpkin," they called me "The Fat Pumpkin". This was the moment in my life when being fat was no longer adorable. My teammates were the first to clue me in. It took about two weeks for "Man, you really stink" to turn into "Hey Fatty, you suck."

Okay, now I understand my orb-ness adversely affects my athleticism. But my circumference has nothing to do with my failed attempts to catch a ball or inability to make contact with every single pitch thrown my way. Clearly, that "fat kid" rhetoric was unnecessary. Since it was tee ball, we eventually started to practice hitting the ball off of said tees. When it got around to my turn, it looked like I was attempting to play tetherball while having a seizure. After many failed attempts and useless taunting, it occurred to my coach that my inability to hit the ball might stem from my inability to actually see the ball. He asked me if I have ever had an eye exam or been considered for glasses.

Truly, that was the last thing I needed. If there is one way to draw more attention to a fat kid, it is by putting glasses on them. You couldn't imagine my glee. A few years later I added braces, which made me one of the few Triple Crown winners of social inadequacy. Amazing. I digress. Though the addition of glasses brought a lot of insult, it also brought the ability of sight. Oddly enough, seeing the ball made it a whole lot easier to hit and catch. And, being a fat kid shrunk an already difficult strike zone to almost nothing. So, I would crowd the plate until I got four balls. Instead of taking the free pass to first base, they would bring out the tee. Once I learned how to put my weight into the ball, I could hit it pretty far. In an attempt at sportsmanship, the rules stated that no matter how far the ball was hit, you were only allowed to advance as far as second base. This was amazing. Excitement abounds. My strategy was defined for the rest of the season:

- Crowd plate

- Get walked

- Hit ball hard

- Don't even bother running because you are only allowed to go to second base anyway

- It's a win-win-win

I loved this plan. Needless to say, the season ended with many doubles, countless treats, and a uniform that was so tight it would have looked better if it were just painted on instead. Scratch that, I have been to New Orleans and there is clearly a weight limit that comes into play on a thread-to-skin ratio. Let's keep those pants on no matter how much muffin top occurs.

For the next year, I did everything I could to prepare for Little League because I knew that as long as I had a reason to leave the house, I would have an opportunity to snack. Who knew that so much adult knowledge could be learned from such a youthful game?

Chapter 2:

Two Wheels On a Huffy vs.

Two Reeboks On a Chubby

With fifth grade on the horizon, my mother and father issued a parental directive that was as influential on my individual development as it was detrimental to my nutritional future. The first step was entrusting my sister and I with the responsibility of not only walking home by ourselves, but also having a key to the back door of our house.

The second step involved me handling a $10 weekly allowance for school lunches and other needs. I got a raise because the price of in-school lunch increased from $1.00 to $1.10. This was one of the greatest things that could have happened to me. I was able to roll the extra $.90 per day into a snacking fund. Think of this as a cell phone minute rollover plan for chubby kids. It's my little version of Initech, minus the stapler.

What mustn't get lost in all of this was my sister's role. Theoretically, she was supervising me until my parents got home. She was in eighth grade and should have had enough good sense to oversee any abuses of such an allowance. But let's be real; she was in the *eighth* grade. While her age suggested she was mature enough to supervise me, her hormones dictated her concern towards which boys she had a crush on. So for all intents and purposes, her fat little brother was left alone to his own caloric devices. Nice.

Snacking aside, I seized the opportunity to stockpile candy and snacks in various hidden locations through the house. No one was the wiser. Vive la resistance!

While I was showing the snack stockpiles a good amount of attention, my waistline was quick to remind me that it too, was ever-expanding. With my stomach continuing to challenge the limits of elasticity, my parents did their best to keep me in line with acceptable fashion trends. They always offered to take me out and suit me up with the flavor of the week jeans and t-shirt brands. I would cordially decline. Sweat pants and baseball jerseys were my uniform of choice. What society does not know or comprehend is that jeans are a torture device to the overweight and under-firm. Let me explain.

First, jeans have a button. This means there is non-elastic resistance pressing into your stomach at *all times*. ALL TIMES!!! It does not move or flex with you in the way that elastic drawstrings do. Rather, it digs into you, ceaselessly reminding you that breathing is slowly becoming an ever-laboring task. Mind you, that's just when you're standing up. When you sit down, well, that's an entirely different story.

Envision someone cinching you into a corset against your will. Then picture them tightening it as though they were trying to gain classified information from you. The resulting pressure makes one sweat even more than carrying the extra weight does. The jeans have an uncanny ability to lift and separate what has become a 36-inch flesh-filled muffin top that cannot be hidden or concealed with any form of dignity. Unless, of course, one has a previously stretched oversized black shirt on hand. Then, there might be a shot. But even then, if the shirt is not stretched out in advance, you end up looking like a sausage. Nobody wants that. To avoid that whole scene, I'd wear a button down shirt in which the final 2 buttons remained open and strategically draped over my waist. Thank you, baseball jerseys.

Second, when you are overweight, your thighs rub together a lot. I mean a lot. Have you ever heard the term thunder thighs? This term was probably created when someone observed a left thigh (warm front) and a right thigh (cold front) rubbing together at such a torrid pace (walking) and assumed the colliding raw flesh would ignite a sound so thunderous that this clever moniker was the only way to properly describe it. I don't know about you, but when my legs are rubbing together, the last thing I need is denim to escalate the thigh-on-thigh action. What I *do* need is the sweet comfort of cotton to sooth my savage thighs. And what better source for cotton than sweat pants? Right? Right!

Though sweat pants kept my National Weather Service thighs at bay, they did very little to impress the ladies and gentleman commonly known as my peers. You see, with middle school on the horizon, people became aware of social positioning. They started to buy into the importance of fashion, and well, my comfort waistband and I never stood a chance. But you know what? It really didn't matter. No matter how badly the world wanted to make fun of my fashion or reject my character, I always had the open arms of my snacks to comfort me. Thanks to that additional $.90, pressure alleviation was just a nickel, dime, or quarter away. You can't always pick who you sit next to in math class, but you can always pick where you find your contentment. As for me, red, yellow, orange, and green Sour Field Kids were my top four. Tom who? MySpace hasn't even been thought of yet.

As successful as I was at lying to everyone else, I was the worst at deceiving myself. Don't get me wrong, I loved my food. But the feeling of social inclusion had no comparison. To know that you are wanted and loved, I cannot think of a greater feeling. Even the insults of people I didn't know were better than the silence of my bedroom. I had no idea I could be surrounded by social opportunity and yet fail to connect with any aspect of it.

In a last-ditch effort to find a place in social hierarchy, I did what any stable-minded adolescent would do. I became an after-school crossing guard. Now before you disagree with my decision, let's think of the benefits of being a crossing guard:

1. I got a really cool badge. I decided to make a little wallet for mine. You know, C.S.I.-style.

2. I got out of school 20 minutes early to ensure prompt arrival at my crossing post. You know the creed: no underclassmen left behind.

3. My post was three feet from Abers.

However, plans don't always go, well, as planned. The teacher liaison for the patrol squad was a chubby popular teacher and my hope was that I would second-hand some cool by associating myself with him. Nope. That theory proved to be flawed. As it turned out, he was creepishly flirty with all the pretty girls and real friendly with all the jocks. Adding insult to injury, my safety satchel didn't fit at all. Not even close. The Hatfields and McCoys were closer to finding peace than the two ends of my sash were to finding each other. I had the largest available and even that one couldn't buckle. Truth be told, that's the real reason my badge wallet was created. I had nowhere else to put it. I was as unpopular with my attire as I was with the kids in school. As luck would have it, people associated those with the responsibility of upholding rules and regulations as snitches.

Snitches were not liked.

Fat kids were not liked.

I was not liked.

In taking the time to evaluate my current situation, I tried to make my quest for popularity as objective as possible. The truth, as I rationalized it, was this: I only had to deal with those people for, at worst, eight hours a day. My calculations would suggest that I had twice as many hours to devote to eating or sleeping or both. At this point, I was beginning to appreciate those options much more than the games of social politics. If all my existence meant to society were fat jokes and taunting, then I would embrace my lack of social status. I would suppress my emotions and drive them so far inside myself that even I wouldn't acknowledge their existence. They lay buried under a myriad of chewy caramel fillings, crunchy roasted peanuts, and most importantly, soft nougaty centers.

While these short-term emotional bailouts were great shots in the arm, they were doing very little for my long-term emotional recovery. The lines between reality and the reality I was creating quickly became blurred. Holding on to fake smiles and good spirits were my best attempts at deflecting any attention towards my blossoming emotional pain and depression. While I was victoriously leading a brilliant dance around my true emotional state, I was clearly losing in terms of girth concealment. What was worse, any other kind of youthful dependence would have been much easier to conceal. If I were a cutter, I would have simply embraced fashions that revolved around long sleeves. The same would have been true for needle-based drugs. If alcohol was my comfort, then I could have developed an affinity for mouth rinse, breath mints, and mindless frat-boy humor. But I was not one of those people. I was merely a fifth grader who weighed 150 pounds. A kid who was less trustworthy around a pan of soft bake snicker-doodles than the Cookie Monster.

I wasn't the only one suffering. My parents were growing more concerned about my physical and mental well-being; they noticed not only my straining emotions, but my straining elastic as well. In an attempt to coyly direct me towards better health, they presented me with a proposition. It went something like this:

Hey son, we've noticed a bunch
of the kids on the block
riding around on mountain bicycles.
They look like they're having fun.
Do you think that's
something you would enjoy?

Wait? No more training wheels?!?
Man....would I ever!
I mean, yes.
Yes, it would be something I would enjoy.

Well, you have proven yourself
responsible with the key to the house
we have given you and we feel

that you can handle the responsibility
of taking yourself to baseball practices.
Well, the practices we can't drive
you to because of work.
Do you feel you can handle
that responsibility?

Oh man, you betcha!
I mean,
I feel worthy of this additional responsibility.

Alright then, it's settled.
We will go out tomorrow
and you can pick out the
bike of your liking.

SSSSSWWWWWEEEEEEEEEEEEEETTTTTTTTTT!
NO MORE TRAINING WHEELS!!!!!!!!
I GET A BIG BOY BIKE!!!!!!
I mean, thank you for this opportunity.

Now, what you have here is classically good parenting.
They took something that was seemingly negative (exercise)
and also necessary (even more exercise) and made it appear fun
and exciting. Also, by asking me questions such as "Would you
like" and "Do you feel," it made me a part of the decision
making process. Statistically speaking, if someone feels
ownership of a situation, they are more likely to participate in it.
Riding the bike would equal more exercise and everyone would
benefit. This is your classic win-win situation.

However… The problem with smart parents is that sometimes, they raise smart kids. Case in point, me. I knew exactly what they were doing with this whole proposition and quite frankly, I didn't care. Do you know why? Playing along with this exercise charade was a small price to pay for the freedom that a bike would bestow upon me. Do you understand the operational radius I was about to acquire?

Last time I checked my telemetry, two wheels on a Huffy cover a lot more ground than two Reeboks on a chubby. Remember, walking for me was a chore. Don't get me wrong, it was well worth the effort to acquire the food; however, that didn't lesson the drudgery of the exercise. But, with a bike, the opportunities became endless! In a single day my coverage area went from one candy store to three convenience stores, a bakery, and a slice-by-slice pizzeria. What once seemed so far away was now within striking distance. Candy will forever hold a fond place in my heart, as one's first love always does.

As I was finally closing that chapter of my life, I was introduced to a friend of whom I would become quite familiar. Her name was Irony. As a lady of the night, Miss Irony does go by several different names: Coincidence, Karma, and Providence. Call her what you may, but for her influence on what happened next, I called her my best friend.

While wrapping up a pick-up baseball game, I overheard some teammates making their lunchtime plans. Always interested in the opportunity for consumption, I asked them what they were talking about.

> *Oh, we were thinking about heading up*
> *to the elementary school to grab some*
> *free grub. We thought about inviting*

you, but we also wanted make sure that
there was enough food for all of us.
So you can see why you weren't invited.

Wow guys, that's some comic genius.
The fat kid likes food.
Thanks for your contribution to society.
However, your personal attacks
do not bother me, for
I have the information I need.

What? Did you whisper something?

No, it was just a sigh from lack of inclusion.

Wait? Did I understand that correctly, a free lunch at
the elementary school for anyone? This seemed too good to
possibly be true. It couldn't be accurate, could it? No, this had
all the signs of a setup. Nevertheless, I kept my distance as I
followed them up the hill. Waiting for them to turn off at any
moment, I took my place behind a tree to observe their next
move. To my surprise, they turned left into a sea of seemingly
hungry faces. Huh?

I guess that made sense because I had never seen the
elementary building that busy when school was not in session.
There was definitely much more activity than normal. So I
nervously approached the window to peer inside. Once I did,
marvelous wonders beheld. As fate would have it, free lunch
summer was not only a reality, but it was happening RIGHT

THEN! But why?

In an attempt to ensure that families were getting proper nutrition over the summer months, the state implemented a two-year initiative that funded free summer lunches for all those families whose residence fell within in the Steel Valley School District zoning lines.

Legalities aside, it was as though the hand of God was pushing my chubby little behind through the pearly gates of mid-summer sloth. For that, blessed be Thy name. The weeks that followed were bliss. Every morning, I would wake up around 10:00 and eat breakfast. Then I waited an hour or so to take a "healthy bike ride" to work off the breakfast I just consumed. Little did my parents know that my planned route would take me right past the elementary school to get my free lunch, sometimes two, if I was lucky.

After that, it was off to the convenience store for a Little Deborah dessert. Public school GEL-OH desserts were terrible, even if they were free. Once the real dessert was consumed and enjoyed, it was a 45-minute walk uphill to return home. Gravity is fun when you can use it to your advantage, but peddling uphill is just more effort than it's worth.

Upon my return home, my mother would greet me with a hug of praise for her baby boy, who was making such a good effort to stay healthy. So proud of the effort in fact, that she would prepare me a special lunch. Grilled cheese, cheesy egg sandwiches with jelly...all of my favorites! Three meals in three hours. I Am Legend.

That behavior carried on all summer long. Throw in a little baseball snacking (in the form of after-game pizza, hot dogs, and snow cones) and my life was becoming more and more complete. My parents, however, still had great concern that their attempts were not working as planned. I gained 10 pounds during summer break and you could see their frustration grow and grow. I had them convinced I was making such an honest effort that they would not think I was sabotaging it.

They never figured that every bike ride included a side route, which lead to a free lunch or two. They were clueless to the skillful web I produced through my above-average creativity, tempered with an incurable adoration for eating. All they could see was their baby boy going out every day, attempting to be active through sports and bike riding. They just couldn't figure out all of the inconsistencies. How, with all of our combined efforts, was no progress being made? They were losing their son to an eating disorder that none of us knew existed.

Chapter 3:

The Dark Ages

BBBBBBBBBBUUUUUUUUUUZZZZZZZZZZZZZZZZZZ!!!!!!!!!!!!!!!!!!

6:00 a.m. The alarm woke me from a fantastic slumber in which dreamland bestowed upon me the mystical key to Pizza Shed City. The magical Leoplurodon had also given me the Golden Pan, which meant that all I had to do was think about a pizza and it would appear. No cost and more importantly, no wait.

BBBBBBBBBBUUUUUUUUUUZZZZZZZZZZZZZZZZZZ!!!!!!!!!!!!!!!!!!

6:15 a.m. Oh come on! I had just received an order of cheesy sticks. What could have possibly been so important that it couldn't wait!?! It was about to be the best PAN-demic ever. Oh dang it! Was that only a dream? It was, wasn't it? But it seemed so real. I swear I tasted the stuffed crust pressed gently upon my lips Sigh.

I dealt with the enormous letdown of false hopes by staring at the ceiling for a couple of minutes. As I wiped the sleepiness from my eyes, I began to ponder just how my first day of middle school would play out. After marinating on that for a moment, I reluctantly rolled out of bed. While passing through the kitchen on my way to the downstairs shower, I was greeted with the familiar aroma of coffee and cigarettes. Such a vivid reminder that yes, indeed, another school year was about to begin.

As the cold water fell from the spout onto my face, I realized that 70% of the school had no idea who I was. They didn't know just how lame, insecure, addicted to food, non-funny, situationally awkward, depressed, fashionably challenged, and socially unstimulating I was. Of course they knew how large I was, but so were John Candy and Chris Farley. I thought to myself, "Those guys are fat and people love them. So Jeremy, this is your opportunity to be "that guy." Go ahead, let people love you because you're fat. Carpe the diem, Rochford! Seize this day, sir, because your life starts now. Yes, yes it does."

I rode that wave of excitement through the rest of my morning routine. While I was planning my entrance, I failed to realize we were already there. As we pulled up, my mother kissed me on the cheek and wished me a great first day of middle school. Most kids would have yelled at their parents for taking away too many cool points with that move. Not me. Not that day. No, I was larger than the image I was about to create.

I stepped out of the car and with a cocky swagger, I proceeded up the walkway. From left to right, I scanned the landscape of social groups. After an initial visual sweep, two groups of *friends* caught my attention. The first group was composed of the cool, older kids from Little League. I figured, why wait until baseball season when we could become friends now? I thought we could get a head start on making fun of those outcasts of which I intended not be a part of. The second group was composed of those very same outcasts I planned to disassociate from. They were the leftovers from not only Little League, but all other sects of life as well.

With my newfound confidence, I headed straight to the older kids' group. Before I could stop walking and make eye contact, I was greeted with, "Hey, here comes a fatty," and "Hey penguin, better slow your waddle down before somebody gets hurt." Needless to say, that did not go as planned. After that reception, there was no need to stop. No need to pass GO, and no need to think about collecting $200 worth of cred points. Nope. I just put my head down and kept walking over to Baltic Avenue to join the rest of the outcast group. It was such a dynamic group of individuals who seemed to fail in all aspects of life. The too fats, too skinnies, too slows. Yep, if there was someone who didn't quite fit in, they fit in there. For better or worse, those were my people.

As the bell rang to usher in another long year, I packed up my insecurities and headed towards homeroom. Upon arrival, we were herded up to the chalkboard in alphabetical order. Once our alphabet was straight, we divided ourselves into rows based upon our last name. Those were our seat assignments for the remainder of the year.

I loathe the first days of a new school year. I hated that even in a new school, with new people, my last name still positioned my seat around girls who knew they were good-looking. Why would I complain about that, you might ask? Trust me, as a pre-teen male, I would have loved to sit around all of these blossoming ladies and had a visual buffet. And If I were thin, I might have gotten away with it. But I was not. I was space-consuming, and because of that, I got awkward stares when people realized they had to sit next to me. My best conclusion is that they felt too close to the "blast zone." Blast zone? Yes, blast zone. Remember, as a fat kid, one of my superpowers was flatulence. Even when I was not the culprit, I still got blamed. Yet another reason I lived in social fear.

I thought to myself, "Come on, Rochford, think positive. What is going on right now that is positive? Think.........about it"........badow, there it was on the wall. It looked like an angel. Our in-class television was broadcasting a program that seemed to be a serious upgrade. There was a new morning news show called Channel One that was actually watchable

While the television had improved, my introduction into middle school was not going as I had hoped. The school year had just begun and I was already being made fun of. I couldn't even make it past the pre-game of standing outside, waiting for the bell. As the day progressed, it did not get any better as my hope for change was relegated to nothing more than an attempt at survival. With the undeniable importance of social positioning, I had no idea how to keep up. Boys liking girls, girls liking boys, and as for me...well.... no one liked me. With all the attention now turning to attraction, my fashion choices were also called into question. Gone were the days of cartoon t-shirts and sweat pants to make way for the era of button down shirts, designer labels, and of course, blue jeans.

Now you know my history with jeans, so I won't even begin to waste your time with my feelings on the matter. What I will waste your time with is the delightful revelation that basketball swoosh pants are equipped with the exact same elasticity and breathability as sweat pants. However, for some reason, they fell completely off of the radar when it came to social persecution. Interesting. Because of that fact, I attempted to reform my image from sloppy into sporty. I know. The irony of a kid so overweight that he is unable to fit into age-appropriate fashion attempting to pull off the sporty image as though it were intentional is pretty overwhelming. I'll give you a moment to take it all in.

As weeks went by and the social politics of the lunchroom settled down, I couldn't help but notice a few ladies now inhabited our lunch table. As it turns out, we gentlemen were not the only ones who were feeling alone and socially outcast. The one thing I loved about adolescent socialism is that it knew no gender bias. Another thing is that it somehow self-perpetuated.

With the addition of young ladies to the lunch table, I found myself pushed even further to the outside of the social circle. I decided to reinvest in an old romance that some hoped I would outgrow. I decided to leave the hope of a new beginning for the hope of what was. The comfort of my beloved. I continued to eat. A lot. After a short while, all hopes of social acceptance had left my psyche and eating was all I could think about.

My life became a series of patterns that all revolved around eating. When I went to bed, I looked forward to waking up because I knew I would be able to eat. When I went to school, I looked forward to lunch because I knew I would be eating. Once I was done with lunch, I looked forward to my walk home because it would consist of the three-point pit stop, which became affectionately known as the "Munhall Hat-Trick."

It started with a local pizzeria named Detories. After a slice or so, my good ol' choo-choo shoes lead me up the street to G & K Bakery. My daily visits with the doughnut lady became as routine as breathing. It was as good for the mind as it was for the wallet: after 3 p.m. the bakery sold discount pastries because they were then considered day-old stock. For me, these

$.25-cent rings of glaze were heaven. The third stop along this walk of champions was Abers. You never forget your first love. It will always cut the deepest. In my case, it did so while remaining the most financially responsible. While other chumps were wasting their allowance on Sorcery: the Gathering cards and Street Brawler tournaments, I was honing my ability to conquer candy mile.

After the .2-mile walk from Abers to my basement, it was time to detox with candy therapy and my 3:15 appointment with Dr. Magnavox. Every single day seemed to be a struggle, but I knew that if I took life in four-hour increments, I would either be sleeping or eating, both of which made life just bearable enough.

As the leaves changed and the holidays drew near, I had only one reflection for those gloomy winter months: was this really all there was to my life? I mean, living in four-hour increments just to make it through the day? What would it have been like to have a real connection with a girl?

For all of the nonsense I thought of for the holiday, there was only one wish I had for Christmas. I wished that God would shed a little grace on me. That He would show me glimpses of something better, something more than the life I was living. It was a holiday season full of hopes and prayers. Kinda. I guess I didn't pray for anything, really. I mean, I prayed in that way where you are half asleep and you ask God for some kind of miraculous change that you are prepared to receive, but never intend to put any work into helping facilitate that change. Yeah, in that way I prayed. It was no surprise that God put as much effort into my social reform as I put into asking Him for it. Just another holiday full of sweaters to sausage and shoehorn myself into.

As the new year turned into another lonely February, I found myself overwhelmed with self-loathing. My eating life was going well, I was girthing to my full potential, but I was still dwelling on the idea of there being more to life than who I was becoming.

It was also around this time that I developed my first school age crush. Rebecca was her name, and ever since the ladies got integrated with the rest of us outcasts, she was the only one who had caught my attention. Rebecca came to our group by way of her advanced scoliosis and the brace that paralleled her spine because of it. She was very, very skinny and I am sure at times when we stood next to each other we resembled the number 10.

To me, it hardly mattered. The fact that she spoke to me at all was enough to set my heart aflutter. I was infatuated with the potential of someone being infatuated with me. The idea of being involved in a relationship that didn't revolve around unrequited love was so foreign. To be honest, I don't even know how our relationship started, it just kind of happened. Observations turned into jokes. Jokes turned to conversations about Nirvana, which then blossomed into young love. Aw. While this may seem like a picture-perfect example of an answered prayer, it opened a whole new set of problems. I quickly came to realize that sixth grade dating in terms of physical boundaries and self-respect didn't leave too many options. It wasn't advanced moral fiber that kept our curiosity at bay. Rather, it was the awkward disposition shared by two people so afraid of being alone that risking romantic progression was worth the stalemate in order to preserve any sustained human interaction. Well, that's how I perceived it.

As it turned out, younger women are just not into stability as much as they are into excitement. I never had a chance. It took just one month of walking her home from school and holding hands while mall shopping for it to become clear that our relationship either needed to be taken to the next level, or taken to the grave. Before I got the hint, my headstone was already prepared. Young love is so fragile, so cruel.

With nothing else to fill my time, I was able to work myself back into Dr. Magnavox's candy therapy sessions. For as tough as it was to say goodbye to Rebecca, it was just as nice to rekindle the warm embrace of the Munhall Hat-Trick. As my after-school candy therapy became as routine as it had been before, the good doctor turned me on to something that I failed to notice. Somehow, Pittsburgh went from a drinking town with a football problem to a three-sport juggernaut as the Penguins wrapped up their second consecutive Stanley Cup win. Penguin mania was everywhere. Even as a Pirates fan, I could not avoid the Penguins on the after-school sports report.

At first, I did my best to snub it. To me, the Pirates were the only Pittsburgh team that mattered. But after a while, the sheer talent of Jaromir Jagr, Mario Lemieux, and Ron Francis were too entertaining to resist. Oh, Ronnie Francis. He was my favorite. I liked Ron because of his ability to produce the same numbers that other stars put up, but for some reason he was always third- or fourth-tier when it came to interviews. The media's concern was with the pretty and flashy players, and if time allowed, then they would interview Francis. I could relate. I felt as though I was blossoming into a fantastic young individual, who had just as much to offer as anyone else, yet, because I had a couple of extra pounds as well as a love for elastic waist comfort, no one wanted anything to do with me. Ron Francis and I, two of the same.

Fueling my infatuation with the sport was the growing ritual of after-school street hockey that had picked up at the end of my street. As it got warmer, I would pass the games while walking home from school. I always wanted to play, but they were the older kids, and I was far from athletic. I already had bad experiences with upperclassmen and organized sports, so the idea of putting myself through that ridicule again was not appealing. But I really wanted to get involved. I really wanted to belong.

I thought to myself, "I know that I don't have a place in baseball, what with all that running. But in hockey, you glide and sit, glide and sit. I can do that. I can skate for a minute and then sit for five. I can do that. I can transition my hand-eye coordination from baseball into hockey. Yeah, this seems perfect. I can become so good at hockey that people wouldn't even notice how large I am. If they do, it's because they can't carry me on their shoulders due to all of the goals I am going to score." I liked this plan. My next step was convincing my parents that this was the best idea for my weight loss goals. Like any mature sixth grader, I presented my interest in hockey as such:

"Mom...Dad! I need skates and a stick! I want to play hockey and if I don't play then I am just going to die. I'm serious mom, I'll just DIE!!!! I REALLY REALLY REALLY need to play hockey. And if this doesn't happen, then I am just going to die! You don't want me to die do you?"

My parents, who must have had their "concern for his health" filters on to override the obnoxious presentation, must have heard the proposal this way:

"Mother, Father, good day. As you know, my current weight has become problematic for all of us and I feel as though hockey will provide me with an outlet to combat it. It might work, it might not. Either way, it will increase my activity level, and therefore is the best option to attack my weight situation at this time. For my safety, I will need to be equipped with a pair of roller blades, a stick, a pair of gloves, and a ball to practice with. Thank you for your time and consideration in this matter."

I'm still not sure exactly how they took it, but the bottom line is that it was successful. By the end of that week, we were in the local sporting goods store purchasing equipment. My plan was to practice on our back patio until I was good enough to impress the older kids with my ability. I needed to build my confidence to know that once I showed them how amazing I was, there would be no reason for them not to let me play. Forced friendship isn't always the best option, but it's better than being alone.

Without any thought to gravitational law and how it worked against misshapen individuals, I put those skates on and had at it. It turned out that physics had at it as well. As soon as I began to roll, I also began to wobble. The wobbling led to shaking, and the shaking led me flat on my back, face up, trying to hold on to whatever breath and dignity I could muster. Whoever said that the bigger they are, the harder they fall, must have envisioned that exact moment. While the stars twinkled, I began to wonder why a helmet was omitted from our shopping list. I laid there for a good 10 minutes, waiting for my head to stop pounding. Once it finally did, I convinced myself that it might be a good idea to pack it in for the night.

The next day in school, I walked around with a look that mirrored an individual who had gas, ready to drop an air-fluffy at any moment. You see, because of how bad my skating tumble hurt, I could not make complete butt-to-surface contact with any of the seating in school. I was on a cheek-to-cheek rotation pattern, which I am sure had all the aforementioned girls nervous. Truthfully, I didn't even care. That was the first time in my life that I worked for something so hard that it hurt. Plus, I could tell people that I was limping due to some sports injury. That didn't work at all. The limp only incited comments about me waddling because I was too fat to walk normally.

As I limped past the daily street hockey game, I noticed that not everyone was wearing skates. Some players were merely running with their stick. I thought to myself, "Wait. So I don't have to punish my backside for the next four months to gain acceptance? I'm listening. What's the cost of such relief? Wait, I would have to run. Hmm. This is tough because of my stance on running. But I also have a stance on pain. Okay, new plan. I'll learn how to shoot first, and then I'll just stand in front of the net to screen the goaltender. No need to run. No need to skate. Just do what I do best, take up space. While I am there, I'll just get the rebounds and score. This plan seemed flawless."

So instead of going home and lacing up my skates every night, I took my inability to shoot and applied it to our garage door. This annoyed the bejesus out of my mother. She loved the fact that her kid was being active; she hated the fact that it came at the expense of chipping the paint and finish off of the garage door. Realizing that a hockey net is cheaper than the time, effort, and cost that would go into repainting the garage door every three months, I received an actual goal to practice on. For the next week, I spent every waking moment that I wasn't in school, eating, or sleeping, shooting hockey. I took it quite seriously. I affixed paper plates in the corners to mimic targets. I spent every evening picking off corners and gaining accuracy.

Now armed with the confidence to hold my own with the older kids, only one question remained: how could I integrate myself into their game? I thought about it for a few days and formed a rational plan in my head. There were two main players who would shoot around after school, about 20 minutes before everyone else showed up. Due to their high school schedule, high school driving ability, and relational housing proximity, they were the first ones to arrive. If I could target just those two individuals and hang around them until everyone else showed up, I would be grandfathered into playing. It was another flawless plan.

I put it to action. As soon as our bell rang, I made a beeline up the hill and headed straight for home. While it was the most difficult part of the plan, I didn't stop for food and I didn't stop for candy on my way home. As I crested the hill just past the elementary school, I slowed down to catch my breath and composure.

Jeremy, this is your shot.
DO NOT MESS THIS UP!
DO YOU HEAR ME!?!

I frightfully listened to my conscience and as I walked past, I stopped to make general conversation.

Hey, what's going on, guys?

Mind you there were only two of them. So I was riding high on some confidence.

Not too much, man.
Just playing some hockey.
You?

Chillin.
Walking home from school.
You know.
Hey, I see you guys play often.
Do you have room for one more?

Sure, I guess so.
We are always looking for a goalie.
What's your name?

Of course, Goalies.
Um.
Jeremy, Jeremy Rochford.

Hey, do you have a sister named Tami?

Yep.

Okay, cool. I know Tami.
I didn't know she had a brother.

Do you have equipment?

Yeah, I've got some.

Okay, cool.
Grab what you got,
we have a chest protector
and some pads over there.

HOLY SNAP! For the first time in seven years, an engineered social plan of mine actually came to fruition. I couldn't believe it. And they didn't even laugh at me. I give my sister an assist on that one. But wait. GOALIE? Again? Come on, I was going to be a scoring superstar, not a defensive backdrop. ARGH! (Angry, non-pirate)

Most people's introduction into peer pressure comes by way of drugs, sex, or alcohol. Not me, my introduction was throwing away everything thing I had planned and worked so hard for just to fit in and play out a standard fat kid stereotype. But still, it was worth it. I spent the next few months playing goal, all the while learning to skate on my own free time.

As I put more effort into skating, my falls became fewer and farther between. However, your common youth rollerblade is not designed to support a 165 pound 11-year-old. The wheels disintegrated under my pressure just as quickly as I could replace them. After seeing the vulcanized carnage, my parents decided it would just be cheaper to upgrade my skate selection. Even that proved to be futile. Those skates lasted about three months until the boots were ripped away from the chassis. The problem was that youth sizes are not constructed with the intent of supporting an adult weight. But, I made due. I had to. I finally had a group that accepted me as much as I wanted to belong. Even if it was only because my presence meant that they weren't the ones standing in front of the pucks and balls being shot at their head.

My parents were definitely supportive of the more active lifestyle. I liked the fact that I had an even better excuse to eat more often. Burning off all those calories left me very depleted. As an athlete, I needed to be fueled and ready! I started doubling up on meals and amped up my snacking to stay sharp. Before I knew it, school was over and summer was upon us. I traded the heartache of young love for the promise of a summer filled with newfound hockey fame. More importantly, I was wrapping my arms even further around an incurable romance that was nothing short of comfortable.

Chapter 4:

Food: The Other Four-Letter Word

At what point does adoration become obsession?
At what point does obsession become addiction?
At what point does addiction become a disorder?
At what point does a disorder become discovered?

At what point does the interwoven master plan of an 11-year-old child become nothing more than shattered stories of youthful folklore? The answer became very clear as I found myself face-to-face with a military-grade scale and the cold tile floor that was my annual school physical.

Even my best deceptions seemed futile as I tried to charm my way through something that was scientifically out of my depth. I proceeded to sweat nervously, trying to read the upside down freehand that was the nurse's script. It was just as confusing as the look of genuine concern paired with disgust coming from her brow.

I thought to myself, "Could it be that my lifestyle of sneaking food and triple sizing meals had finally caught up with me? Impossible. Kids my age are smoking, drinking, and experimenting with their bodies. There is no possible way my feel-good drag of day-old doughnuts and chocolate frosting could even compare. How dare she judge me like that? What gives her the right? She's overweight herself. How ironic is this? She's the one who is supposed to set a professional example.

What terrible hypocrisy!

OH NO! What if she brings my parents into this? She has every authority to do just that. She would probably do it just to spite me. Why, lady nurse, why? I see your thighs pouring over your knee-highs. I know that you are just like me. "

If you have followed the story so far, you know that my parents were very aware of my weight problems. They believed they were feeding me "healthy," weight-conscious meals. However, they had no idea how methodical my behind-their-back eating had been. I created a phantom perception of their helpless baby boy working so hard to lose weight through controlled diet and athletic participation, but with little avail. I played on the emotions my mother felt when she went to Weight Observers. Having struggled with weight herself, I knew she was sympathetic.

But sympathy and emotion are thrown out the window once scientific evidence is presented. I wondered, " What if the nurse calls me out by playing the health professional card, and puts my stories to the test? What if she calls my REAL doctor to get his opinion on this? Surely he will want to conduct some form of test for absolute clarity. This is not good! This is not good at all!"

The rest of the day, I paced around the halls like a defendant awaiting judgment. Once I arrived home, I quickly realized there was a verdict. My parents had spoken with our doctor and based upon the results of my school physical, he wanted to run a few tests. He was curious to see if there might be other reasons my weight wasn't coming off. He was thinking science and I was thinking shenanigans. Either way, my future was not bright.

I did what any normal kid in my situation would do. I thought of every single lie that I possibly could. I took those lies and dissected their scenarios in my head as though I were writing the playbook for the Super Bowl. Try as I might, none of my tomfoolery seemed to get the upper hand on science. For once in my life, I had finally met my match.

Why was this a big deal, you may ask? Let's put this in perspective. A thyroid test to a food addict is like a drug test to a user. They know that their urine isn't clean, but they still try to figure out some plan to have the test results come back negative. There was an astronomically low chance of beating the system. With such bad odds against me, I expected to face the consequences of my actions.

As the realization of this set in, I could think of only one final course of action: prayer. I prayed in advance for whatever providence the Lord would give me. I prayed so hard that my sister thought I had turned Gregorian. I prayed that our car would break down on the way to testing. I prayed that God would allow me to wake up with a super-sonic metabolism to lose the weight. Above all, I prayed that God would allow me to have an actual medical condition. I prayed so hard that there would be something extremely wrong with me.

I even bargained with God. Growing up Catholic, I remember learning two things from Catechism, God likes to have his fish on Fridays and that all sins are forgivable if you work hard enough. So I swore up and down that if he would not expose me for the addict that I was, then I would tithe all of my allowance to the church. On top of that, I promised that my altar boy-ing would be excellent and free of charge.

Caught you off guard with that one didn't I? Yes, I was

an altar boy. While it has no other relevance to the rest of the story, I mention it to explain my sole motivation for becoming an altar boy: Father Gurdous offered me a king-sized bag of Hershels Minis. Basically, I sold my Sundays for a bag of discount chocolate.

I did everything short of sacrificing a fattened calf in order to get God's attention, but alas, I didn't. The day of the test came as quickly as it went. Fortunately for me, the lag time between the blood draw and the corresponding lab results allowed me to create several forgiveness pleas for when they would be needed. I practiced my speeches and decided to make an actual attempt at dieting. I figured that if I could lose some weight and show my parents success was attainable on my own accord, and then maybe I would have some bargaining power at the time of the verdict.

My commitment lasted two days. I just couldn't take it. There was too much physical exertion with not enough eating for me to stay true. Once again, I found myself praying that God might show me some pity. I sat with a telltale heart as I waited for the day that a singular blinking red light would ruin life as I knew it. The day that I saw the answering machine blinking crimson DANGER, I relinquished myself to the basement for one last moment of splendor. I wonder if this is how an inmate on death row feels, so pensively alive for no real reason.

As I stared at a blank television screen, I heard my mother enter the house. Her footsteps slowed as she approached the answering machine. From the basement I could hear a message, but I couldn't quite figure out what it was saying. I had every hope that it was my uncle calling to check in. In my heart, however, I knew what that message was about. My only wish at that point was this; that I had enough foresight at the time to erase the message before she listened to it. It's the story of my life, always one step behind. Once my mother immortalized the message in digital static for my father's review, she progressed feverishly to the top of the stairs, where she proclaimed:

After dinner we need to speak with you.
Don't you dare go anywhere!

Um, Okay.
What are we going to talk about?

Oh, you'll find out.

To an adolescent, there is nothing worse than an incomplete threat. You know some form of punishment is coming, but you don't know exactly what it is for. One flaw of the human condition is the rate at which parents forget the shenanigans they got away with when they were their kid's age. What makes them think for a second their children are incapable of pulling off the same things they did in their youth, is beyond me. But yet, far too often, they forget. This ignorance opens the door for children to get away with so much.

Because children are so successful at deception, they can develop a superiority complex. That's why the incomplete threat is so dangerous. In the complex infrastructure of the adolescent mind, there are a multitude of schemes being planned that most adults have NO IDEA are even conceivable. So when the youth finally get caught doing something, there is very little time to prepare a counter defense. They can't say just anything. What happens if the counterpoint they conjure up has nothing to do with what they are getting in trouble for? Well, then they have just admitted vicarious guilt to something that wasn't even on the docket. Now all of a sudden, the adults are winning by two. You can't set yourself up like that. So when one of those "we need to talk later" statements presents themselves without a clear reason, it is completely unnerving.

As for me, I knew exactly what we needed to talk about. Not only was I well aware of the problem, I was also well aware that I was defenseless. And go figure, God had failed me. I have no terminal disease. As I turned on the TV to drown out my heavy breathing, I began to wonder what normal people my age were doing. Drugs, sex, alcohol? I had to assume I'm not the only one giving their parents premature gray hair.

But what I really don't understand is how every other form of self-mutilation is taken seriously, but when I impose diabetes upon myself, society finds it funny. Not only that, they make movies about how funny the limitations of the obese are. You always see after-school specials on teen pregnancy and drunk driving, but some how overweight behavior is comical. Could you imagine the media backlash if Hollywood made a feel-good comedy based around the life of a cutter? Cable news wouldn't even know where to start. But somehow, a Scotsman with an incurable desire to digest infants turns my condition laughable. I guess in terms of concern, wrists are more important than waistlines.

My concentration broke as I heard the closing of the front door. My father was home. Upon hearing the message, he stormed to the top of the basement stairs. As he opened the door to yell down, my mother interrupted him by saying:

Bob, he already knows.

My father still threw in *"After dinner!"*

      As our meal was being served and consumed, the tension at the table became so thick you could cut it as though it was the next course. The whole time I was eating, my parents traded glances amongst their plate, me, and then each other. But it always came back to me. Their movements were so repetitious they looked choreographed. I couldn't tell exactly what was going on in their minds, but I felt as though they both wanted to jump across the table and ring my neck for all the lies I had told them. Tempting as it might have been for them, it never happened. Aside from the legal ramifications, my sweaty secondary chin would have proven difficult to complete any kind of asphyxiating maneuver. As the meal concluded, my sister was excused to her room as "we'll talk about it later" had arrived.

So the doctor called today.
You want to know what he said?

That there was a problem?

Oh, there is a problem alright.
He said that the test came back negative
and that your thyroid is in perfect working order,
leaving one of two options.
Either you are a medical enigma or
you have been lying to us this whole time.
Since we have the blood tests to prove
you are nothing special to the world of medicine,
all that is left to conclude is that
you have been lying to us.

As the anger and volume of my father's voice grew, he started to creep closer and closer to my face. My mother, being the angelic voice of reason, reminded him to calm down. He obliged.

So. Do you want to come clean?

I did, oh how I did. All I wanted to do was run into my father's arms and act like a child again. No more scheming infrastructures. No more deception. I hadn't thought like a child my own age for so long. It was always one lie upon another, and all I wanted to do was have it stop. I threw myself at the mercy of my parents and started to cry. I pleaded my case with the difficulties of growing up. I stated over and over that being overweight is the worst obstacle to live through.

Part of my breakdown was a guided tour around the house where I revealed to them all the places in which food was hidden. I was done resisting. I was mentally drained and emotionally dead. After the great housecleaning of stockpiled food, my parents sat me down and administered their punishment. No more allowance. No more freedom. No more lies. The reality that I fought so hard to create now lay just as shattered as my adolescence. Once the emotion of the situation wore off, I found myself once again missing the comfort that food had consistently provided. My opportunities to indulge were now whittled down to nothing.

The closest I came to self-medicating was my indulgent relationship with a tablespoon laden with peanut butter. I found that even through watchful eyes, a tub of anything is difficult to inventory. As part of my rehabilitation, all consumption was to be monitored by both parental units on a meal-to-meal basis. I even got to experience the joys of Weight Observers. "How many points are allotted for my happiness? Not enough," I thought.

I hated my life. I wished things would go back to the way they were. Even hockey lost its appeal. I would rather head straight home from school, do my homework, and attempt to fill the vacancy that food had left behind with B-rate television syndication.

Just as my life was becoming a black rain cloud emo anthem, something magical happened. Upon completion of what is now known as penitence row (without the means to fund the Munhall Hat-Trick, my walk home had been reduced to nothing more than exercise), I huffed though the basement door like I had so many times before. Being a disenfranchised youth, I took great pleasure in banging and throwing things down in a display of unhappiness. This was before iPods, scream metal, and earphone seclusion became the desired choreography of youthful angst; Remember, I'm old school.

This fateful day, I somehow altered the trajectory at which I normally throw my book bag. What resulted was a grandiose overshooting of the bags usual resting place. Upon its decent, the bag clipped the edge of the cushion, causing it to become airborne. My first reaction was, "Fantastic, when this thing lands I am going to have to lift and tuck just so I can bend over to pick it up. This is going to suck."

As I weebled over to the cushion, however, a shimmer of hope caught the corner of my eye. "What is this?" I thought to myself. I took a second glance. Nickels, quarters, dimes! There had to have been at least $4.00 in change there! I threw off the other cushions in anticipatory joy. "Oh yes!!! Oh sweet yes!!!" I exclaimed at the top of my lungs. All of that money and not a single person knew it was there! No one would be the wiser. I ran upstairs to do the exact same thing to the living room couch. I threw aside the cushions with gleeful anticipation. Be still my beating heart. There was an extra $2.00 in that one! HALLLEELLLLUUUUJJJJAAAAHHHH!!

Once my chins were done harmonizing Handel's Messiah, I thought to myself, "Wow, this has turned out to truly be a great day." I was so excited that I literally did not know what to do with myself. It was as though I was on national TV and they just announced that I was the next American Idol. Could you imagine that? What if they fused an annual hotdog eating contest with the sass and pizzazz of non-relevant judges? Now that would be a spectacle. Almost as must-see as what was occurring right then. I'm just glad that I was not a tiny puppy. If I were, I probably would have peed a little.

With out further ado, I jumped on my bike and rode down to the convenience store. It must have looked like something straight out of NASCAR. I was a restrictor plated cliché and I was drafting a phantom on the final lap. That phantom was sugar. I chased it until the checkered flag fell over CoStop's convenience store. Before I knew it, my bike hit the ground, and I was through the door.

Upon entering, I cased the scene for a good 15 minutes. I wanted to take it all in and consider every caloric option carefully. The untrained eye might have assumed I was about to steal something. But, this wasn't the pacing of a thief. It was the pacing of an anticipatory family reunion. Part of me was compulsive and wanted to binge. The rational side was well aware of how temporary these finances could be, and wanted to plan accordingly.

The compromise was one king-sized candy bar today, then a .25 cent snack cake each day for the duration of the money. As I walked my bike up the hill, (citing the obesians' disdain for non-beneficial gravity) my heart was aflutter.

Upon arriving back home, I took steps to ensure that my provisions would last as long as possible. Though most of my food hiding places had been compromised, I had left one storage apparati conveniently overlooked. It was an old dresser which my aunt had gifted me. The top flipped up and doubled as a vanity. The intended functionality was to store jewelry in the little compartments, and then conceal it as the top flipped down. In the good old days, those jewelry compartments were far too small for snack concealment. The attempted storage left nothing but a trail of crushed and distorted snackage in its wake. However, the compartments were aptly sized for all forms of money.

The resurrection of my eating habits made me feel like a new man. I had a swagger restored to my step that only yesterday seemed so distant. The relief of having at least one of the trinitative aspects of the Munhall Hat-Trick restored to my life was more than enough to resurrect my walk home. Oh doughnut store, I'm glad I chose you! To some, you may have only been a stale afterthought, but to me, you were heaven. If cardboard was glaze-able, I would have eaten it.

My days were happy but my weeks were growing long. Try as I might, I couldn't prevent the cash flow from drying up. My coins were running low and my couches were becoming barren. Knowing what I was on the verge of, I grabbed whatever coins I could find and headed for the park. It was time to have an emergency planning session between myself, Dr. Zepper, and Mr. Averagebar. Little Deborah moderated. As we sat and planned our hearts out, no one seemed to have any real ideas to create a viable revenue stream. All I could get out of them was a combination of 23 other ideas and stories about some amusement park in central Pennsylvania. Even Deb was coming up small. As my strategy session drew to a close, I disposed of my brain trust accordingly. Their ideas were bad, but at least their body of work was tasteful.

I walked a few steps and began to kick some rocks around in the hopes it would inspire a grandiose idea. It didn't work, but it did attract my attention to the glimmer of hope that lay before me on the ground. As I got close enough to realize what it was, I found myself caught in an imperfect moment of clarity. Who would have known that this reflective piece of litter would be just the opportunity I needed? The garbage I speak of was the discarded wrapper from a package of baseball cards.

My parents, on numerous occasions, suggested that I take up a hobby of some sort to divert my mind from my desires to eat. The epiphany I had was to combine the best of both worlds. How so? My parents wanted to be supportive. They would buy into this new approach to curb my dietary habits and invest in the building of a baseball card collection. Along the way, I could siphon any cards of worth and pawn those off to the highest bidder. I could then take a portion of the income generated from the valuable cards and replace it with a card or so of minimal worth. Then I could take the profit and invest in the eating habit I desired. With that system intact, the volume of my collection increased as did the side account designed to afford my caloric needs.

Genius. Welcome back, Jeremy Rochford. The game needed you.

At what point do emotions cause worry?
At what point does worry become concern?
At what point does concern become action?
At what point does action become hope?
At what point does hope become lost?

Chapter 5:

Letters From the Edge

With lady luck somehow fancying my attention, I let her indulge. Why not? She and I had made quite the pair lately. Not only did she help me overcome all of the obstacles placed between food and I, she also allowed me become smarter in the process. Now that's love. The kind that makes you want to become a better person. Even deeper than that, it's the kind of love that makes you want to become a superhero! Incrediboy, now that's a superhero!

While lady luck acted as my sugar mama, both figuratively and literally, I took the time to relax and enjoy the fruits of our amazing courtship. As my mind began to wander from snack cake joy to nougat-covered highways, I somehow found myself in a head-on collision with reality. Part of the collateral damage was realizing that my baseball card scheme was not so much a means to an end as it was a temporary stopgap. If I was ever going to sustain my eating habits, then a long-term financial strategy was needed. But at that age, how could I diversify? Think, Rochford, think...I had already implored the hobby side of my parent's generosity, what other form of their concern had I yet to exploit?

Think about it...think about it...what would a genius superhero do in a situation like that? It's not like it's rocket science or something. Well, no, it's not. Hmm...wait for it...wait for it.... and...SHAZAM! There it was. I should have thought of that earlier! All I had to do was manipulate my disparaging social standing. Clearly, standard adolescent development called for me to put myself into social situations. My father was a psychologist, he would understand that. Furthermore, seeking out social interaction would get me out of the house. The further I was from the house, the further I was from caloric control. I liked that. I liked that a lot.

So then, what was the plan? Well, what is the standard antidote for pre-teen boredom and adolescent angst? Movie theaters and shopping malls, of course! Alright. I scheduled my parents' driving responsibilities around mall trips and movie times, which enabled me to bait and switch the appropriated finances. They were convinced that the money they had given me was going to pay for an inflated price of a current movie; however, my friends and I were actually going to the $1.00 second run movies. The money saved on ticket prices allowed me to afford the concessions that were otherwise unattainable. Combining $3.00 from the baseball card empire with the additional $6.00 my parents had given me then afforded me the large movie combo. Why the large combo? Because the large combo is the only size that offers free refills. Silly, you should have known that.

With my parents unknowingly diversifying my portfolio, I was able to seek out other opportunities. While I say seek, I think it was more likely the guiding hand of my lovely lady luck directing me. One day, as I was going into my parents' room to get a new tube of toothpaste (it's a long story as to why my parents' room held all things hygiene, we can discuss this later), I recognized an opportunity which I had never noticed before. While exiting the closet with minty fresh reinforcement in hand, I noticed a random change jar located next to my mother's sewing machine. I saw the layer of dust that had formed on the top of it and thought, "This looks as though it has never been emptied." I put it on my radar and after two weeks of compiling dust and not interest, I figured it was time to make a withdrawal. Nothing too drastic, a quarter here and a quarter there, you know, just enough.

With the success of this endeavor, I wondered what other opportunities were waiting for me under car seats, couch cushions, and even in junk drawers. All those places garnered such success that my lady directed me into further diversification through my sister's fundraising. Somewhere along the way though, the inner-household deception just wasn't enough for me. The sensation of getting away with schemes became as good of a feeling as eating the food that resulted from them.

The lines were becoming blurred as to which phenomenon was fueling which. Truthfully, I really didn't care, as long as it continued. But where do I go from here? Who could I take from next? How about the places I was already going to buy food from? I was already there as a patron, so, a few juvenile shenanigans wouldn't be the end of the world.

Realistically, if society had embraced a comic strip about the menacing hijnks of a young boy my age, then sneaking a pack of baseball cards here and a candy bar there shouldn't be that bad. It's not like I was shooting a dog with a slingshot or anything. Besides, it's not really stealing if it's for the needy. I liked to think of myself as a modern day Robin Hood. I took food from those who have blessed metabolisms and used it to feed my less fortunate one.

After many successful offenses, I found that taking the

food directly was no longer an option. Chocolate melts and snack cakes get crushed. Have you ever attempted to salvage a crushed Twinkle or a melted anything bar? Let me tell you, it is never a positive eating experience. Nope, it's best to stick with taking the baseball cards from convenience stores to sell them at the flea market.

But why stop there? Why not seek out every opportunity? When we had dinner delivered, my mother would have me go to her purse to get the money to pay the guy, and then place the change back in her purse. Well, it never dawned on me before because it never mattered, but she never counted the change I returned. Intrigued by the potential, I started paying attention. I noticed she never kept tabs on her money. How could I pass that up?

I observed long enough to feel confident that I would not get caught. I didn't want to be obvious, so I figured I would start small. I waited until she came home from bingo or from the flea market to grab a couple one-spots. I didn't want to go for a ten or twenty because I felt the higher amounts might raise a few questions. A dollar or two, however, could easily be lost in the shuffle of an early morning flea market hunt, or possibly given as an unaccounted tip after a long night of bingo.

I plotted out my plan and attacked. I grabbed $3.00 out of a wad of one-dollar bills. As I went upstairs to hide my treasure, a rush of adrenaline poured over me like I had never felt before. Closing the door behind me, I lifted up the top of the dresser to add my take to the rest of the portfolio. Upon shutting the dresser, I was overwhelmed by a feeling of disassociation. I was watching myself become something I couldn't stop.

As my hand pulled away from the dresser, my heart dropped as I realized that I had just stolen from my mother. Petty theft from local merchants is one thing, but to steal from the one who brought you into this world is, well, beyond words. I went to open the dresser to take the money and return it rightfully, but I couldn't. My mind told my arm to move, but my arm resisted. It was as though the will to do right was overshadowed by the will to establish success.

I threw myself onto the bed and stared at the ceiling. I convinced myself that my actions were not intended to hurt anyone; they were merely a means to an end. Before I knew it, I was asleep. My life was becoming a nightmare and I wasn't sure if I was sleeping or awake. Once I realized how far into this I was, it was too late to stop. I was already buried. My successful deception had evolved into a house of cards. I knew that if I removed one level of falsity, the rest of the intertwining structure would collapse around me.

Why wouldn't they just let me eat what I wanted? This could all have been avoided if they would have just fed me like I had asked them to. I'd been in nutritional purgatory for far too long and I would do whatever it took to not go back.

While all this was occurring, the school year at hand was coming to a close. On tap for the Rochford crew that summer was a quaint getaway. My parents planned a relaxing week-long trip to the Sarasota and Siesta Keys regions of sunny Florida. It was designed to be the perfect family getaway. My parents, being the loving people that they are, wanted to encourage my fondness for baseball by surprising me with tickets to Sarasota's minor league team. Well, okay, the tickets were for the family. But let's be honest, they were purchased with me in mind. The point is that it was amazing. We were able to meet all of the players and get everyone's autographs. I even caught a foul ball and received a broken game bat as a memento. It was truly the best experience of my life. My parents did all of this for me. Their kindness is what made all of my deception so much more repulsive. I never wanted to hurt anyone, I only wanted to eat. I wish they could have seen that.

Another part of the vacation was to be spent visiting my uncle, who lived about an hour away from where we stayed. Through talking with my mother, he knew that I had a collection of baseball cards and couldn't wait to let me see his. Once we got to his house, it was the first thing I noticed. His collection was massive! It wasn't just scrub and no-name cards either. No. These cards were GOOD ones. Beam Team Good! It was a collection filled with tons of inserts, rookies, and top dollar stars alike.

Now, with the successes of my other portfolio endeavors, I figured that spreading the family wealth would be easy. His collection was so massive; I figured that he wouldn't notice if a few cards were missing. So, I took my chances. I grabbed as many inserts and rookie doubles as I possibly could without looking obvious.

My plan was to get back to the hotel and resell them as quickly as possible. Which, as a side note, is the worst thing you could do. Let's be real, it's one thing to steal and have to shamefully give back whatever you took. It goes to an entirely different level when you steal and have to somehow replace what you have pawned. So if you are planning on stealing, just keep that in mind. You know what, second thought, just don't steal at all. Moving on.

If there was one convenience of being fat, it was the unshakable awkwardness that always seemed to a pre- and post-cursor of my existence. Somehow, this gravitational pull of awkwardness makes extraordinarily awkward situations seem normal. Confusing, I know. This is probably why there are no theorems based around it.

As we headed for the hotel, I was already making mental preparations to sell the cards. The true quandary was how? I was in such unfamiliar territory and running out of ideas when my family made a stop for some souvenir shopping. As I was making my way to the gift shop, I noticed a baseball card store across the plaza. How convenient. Lady luck, I didn't know you were coming along on this vacation, you naughty girl! Seeing this as my only opportunity, I convinced my parents that I didn't need to look at another round of discount Florida t-shirts. Realistically, I was never going to wear one of those shirts, if for no other reason than the giant screen-printed sun stretched across the front of it. The last thing I needed was to wear an XXL Floridian sun to confuse those I have already eclipsed.

So I grabbed my cards from the van and went to the baseball card store. I walked through the door with one thing on my mind: **SELL THE EVIDENCE**.

Well hello there young sir,
how may I help you?

I want to know if you are interested in
buying some baseball cards.

Okay, well let's see what you got here.

Wow...that's quite a collection.

Yeah, I have an uncle who likes me a lot,
 I just have no use for them.

*You're telling me. So what brings
you down this way?*

Oh I'm on vacation, we are visiting an
uncle who lives in the area.

Really, what's his name? I might know him.

Oh no, you probably don't.

By this time I was starting to tremble and sweat even
more so than your typical obesian in the hot Florida sun. I could
see in the clerk's eyes that he wasn't quite buying my story. He,
unlike most people, seemed to know the difference between
overweight awkward and up-to-something awkward. So he
started asking me more probing questions.

Come on, try me.

Um....ah....Theodore Rogus.

*Oh Theo, I know Theo.
And he just gave these to you?
Are sure that he wants you to sell these?*

Um, you know what?
On second thought, I'm just going to keep them.
Thank you for your time.

With the quickness of a lifted eyebrow, I walked away from the counter and out through the door. It was all that I could do to keep my legs from collapsing under the stress that now inhabited my entire body. As we drove back to the hotel, a full body migraine accompanied by its obnoxious friend queasy decided to get involved with my downward spiral. I stared out the window until we arrived.

I walked up the stairs to our hotel room, and just as I was attempting to lie down, the phone rang. Once my mother picked up the phone, it became quite clear I was about to become the receiving end of many sirens. Anytime someone listens more than they speak, good news surely will not follow. Her face turned from carefree to confused, bypassed understanding, and headed straight towards angry. All I could audibly decipher was a choir of ah-has and okays, which seemed to contrast the mounting sniffles and cracking voice. Even though her hands were shaking, she did her best to compile a list of what I assumed were the missing cards.

I thought to myself as she hung up the phone, "Is this how it really ends, on a vacation, of all places?" With the compassion of a saint, my mother summoned me forth to give me one final attempt at an honorable surrender. She asked if there was anything I would like to say or maybe confess to? By this point I was so paralyzed by fear, I couldn't even form words, just blubbering ramble. Accepting that as my plea, she asked me to bring her my collection of cards. As she went through them, she began to align the cards with the list of those missing. With each line that was crossed off, I received a corresponding sigh and stare of disappointing disbelief. Her breath was heavy and only interrupted by the pause of sniffles and held-back tears.

Upon completion of the list, my mother instructed me to wait in the car. I sat there for what seemed to be an eternity. I watched through the windshield as my mother explained to my father what the phone call was about. I waited even longer as she did her best to calm him down. Acting as unwillingly composed as possible, my parents both entered the car and we drove up the Florida interstate to return the stolen cards to their rightful owner.

There was no radio, no conversation, not even a justified swearing rant. The only audible movement was the out of time beating coming from a mother's broken heart. The silence felt more like the mourning of their son's innocence than it did punishment. Conceivably, this was the most embarrassed my mother had ever been in her life.

My uncle was very gracious as we returned the stolen property. Upon our return to the car, my mother turned to me with bloodshot eyes. With the force that had oppressed multiple tears she mustered in a low register, *"How could you?"* She repeated it over and over again as though I had momentarily broken her thought process. *"How could you?"* I had no answer.

As my mother began to cry, my father seemed just as unstable. The husband inside wanted nothing more than to grieve and console his wife for the embarrassment she felt, while the father inside wanted nothing more than to sternly punish his ever-so-deserving son. For the first time in my life, my parents had no idea what to do next. They had never experienced disappointment of this magnitude. My sister, four years my senior, was an exemplary honors student. She was a social butterfly that enjoyed community service and band auxiliary. While she had her own imperfections, they were far from criminal.

Then there was me, the son. The black sheep of the family who became so addicted to food consumption that thievery and deception became as common as breathing. Why did this happen? How did this happen? I was given every opportunity my sister had. Instead of using my abilities for the benefit of others, I used them for the deception of others. What is a family to do in a situation like this?

No one ever tells that side of the story, the one in which the family members of the addicted person suffer just as much as the member who is afflicted. How many mothers cry themselves to sleep while they wonder what they did wrong? How many fathers punch a hole through a wall to make sure their true anger doesn't become misdirected? How many siblings face the social fallout of their sibling's dysfunction?

The next day would stand paramount as the most awkward day of my life. Not foreseeing any of this, we still had tickets to one final baseball game. Figuring there was a less likely chance of a scene in public and not wanting to waste honestly earned money, my family forged on with smiles that were as plastic as the seats we were sitting in. What should have been a final memory of our great family vacation was reduced to nothing more than a wrestling match between emotional restraint and public etiquette.

The drive back to Pennsylvania was more of the same,

tolerable at best. Everyone's mindset was to get home and back to normality as soon as possible. There were a few times I almost peed myself, however, no one found it necessary to be overly accommodating. Aside from gaining urinary control, the trip afforded me plenty of time to reflect on my actions. My mind balanced thoughts of all my prior wrong doings as well as viable ways of killing myself.

In that moment, I wasn't sure what would happen once we returned home. All I knew was that I never wanted to cause my mother that amount of pain again. I couldn't imagine I would have ever done something so unforgivable. For the next few hours, I pondered numerous ways to efficiently cease my existence. I wasn't sure how I wanted end myself, but I knew I didn't want it to be an ordeal. I did not want to leave a giant mess for my parents to clean up. Whatever I chose, I felt that it had to be concise. I didn't want to construct some half-hearted plan that would leave me paralyzed or brain-dead. No, quick and clean, that way I would never hurt anyone ever again.

As I shifted my gaze from the side window to the front of the car, I caught a glimpse of my mother's face. While a silent movie of suicidal completions resonated through my mind, I wondered what she might be thinking. I wondered if she wished she never had me. I wondered if she would ever look at me the same way. I wondered if ending my life would cause more problems for her than living it. I had nothing.

As I looked at my mother, I began to realize that ending my life would for all intents and purposes, end hers as well. How would her heart beat once her love-to-child ratio was forever off by one? If petty theft drove her to react the way she had, how would my suicide make her react? Surely she would convince herself that my demise was her fault, therefore never forgiving herself for it. That's not fair to her, that's not fair at all. Plus, it would completely miss the objective of my suicide in the first place, which was no more pain. Once again, I had nothing. None of this was anyone's fault but my own, and since that was the case, if I was going to be the one living with it, then I should probably be living.

The mental struggle forced me into a migraine-induced sleep coma, and before I knew it, we were back in Pennsylvania. Once I contributed my part of the unpacking, I went up the stairs and straight to bed. The next day, my parents called a meeting for the three of us. They sat me down and with equal looks of disbelief asked me:

> *How does this happen?*
> *I mean, what could you*
> *possibly have to say?*

After the tears, heartache, and utter embarrassment I caused, I felt the least I owed them was an explanation. To the best of my ability, I explained everything I had done since the moment I was placed on dietary restriction. I confessed that the entire baseball card collection was a scam. It was nothing more than a filtration system used to generate income. I proceeded to explain that the money it had produced wasn't enough to keep up with the amount of food I wanted to consume. With very few options, I turned to stealing. At first it was baseball cards to pawn for money. Then it escalated into candy bars from my sister's fundraising kits. Finally, it was straight cash money.

I tried to explain that before I realized what I was doing, I was already in far too deep. I also explained that it was never my intention to become a thief or to succeed in deception, I just wanted to eat. I felt that I had no other options. I had no income. They were controlling my meals at home. All I wanted was for life to be the way that it used to be.

My parents were speechless. The looks on their faces read of disbelief. To know that my efforts and intelligence could have been used for things so much greater than self-destruction left my parents silent.

Without any emotion, my parents sent me to my room. They told me to stay there until the next day. As I sat there in solitude, I was overcome by two completely different emotions. The first was utter repentance as all of my deceptions kept replaying in my mind. However, the second emotion was completely different. As I sat amongst the ruins of strife and broken hearts, I somehow felt justified for every action. For as much pain as I caused, it could have all been avoided had they only let me eat the way I wanted to eat in the first place. Righteousness and remorse battled for control until mental exhaustion finally claimed triumph with slumber as the reward.

Upon waking for breakfast the next morning, my parents once again held council:

Jeremy. We are done fighting you. We have tried everything we can possibly think of to not only help you lose weight, but to also help you realize that you are physically damaging yourself. But, even with our efforts, you just don't seem to care. You don't. The tragedy in all of this is that until you do, we have to wonder what lengths you are willing to go to avoid our direction. I mean, we put you on a diet and you turn into a thief. What next? How far are you going to take this? Things that we never thought you were capable of doing, you have done. We don't want to even fathom what you would consider doing if we pushed you even more. Jeremy. We cannot live your life for you. Until you want this to stop, then nothing we can force upon you is going to help. All we can do is hope and pray that you realize sooner rather than later that you truly are killing yourself. So, here you go. Is this what you want to hear? Jeremy, we give up. No more yelling, no more diets, no more fighting. Eat whatever you want. You win.

Chapter 6:

If You Fake a Smile Long Enough, You May Convince Them It Belongs

"Oh no," he thinks as his head leaps from the pillow.

"Oh no," he hears the familiar hum of a diesel engine resonating through the window.

"Oh no," he ponders as the brakes squeal to stop for every child in sight.

"Oh no," he thinks violently as the anticipation of those children get louder.

"Oh no," is the constant backdrop as he knows he cannot miss another opportunity.

"Oh no," if he does miss this opportunity, surely he will be walking.

"Oh no," the clock is teasing him because he is already running late.

"Oh no," where are his shoes?

"Oh no," where are his pants?

"Oh no," he thinks as he begins to stumble down the stairs.

"Oh no," the front door is locked!

"Oh no," he huffs under his breath as he runs out the door.

"Oh no," it's already too late, what was once so promising is now an evanescent trail of exhaust and fume.

"Wait, wait!" he yells with his arms outstretched as though it was fourth and one with no time on the clock and this was the pinnacle of his existence.

"Oh no!" The vehicle shows no sign of slowing.
"Oh no!" All the children have the ability to stop this.
"Oh no!" They choose to do nothing but mockingly point.
"Oh no!" They have now decided to laugh as well.
"Oh no!" Defeat has slowly crept in.
"Oh no!" Another opportunity slips through his pudgy little fingers.

Most children have nightmares about missing the bus that takes them to and from school. Not I. My greatest fears included a summer day without a frozen delight, as oversleeping had once again allowed the ice cream truck to escape un-Rochforded.

What is this?

What?

This. The whole ice cream truck bit.
Why is it here?

You don't like it?

I never said I didn't like it,
but I will say it's not relevant.

Huh?

You almost killed yourself last chapter,
and now you're cracking jokes?
It just doesn't fit at this point of the story.

I know.
Sometimes I just find it
easier to laugh at my problems,
rather than address them.

I think you owe your readers a little more than that.

I know, but understand my point of view. I just broke my parents. I pushed them so far past the brink of frustration that they gave up. Fearing my greater safety, they felt it was a better option to withdraw parental direction from my eating habits. Don't get me wrong, this was an epic victory for my appetite. But, I never considered the effects my actions would have on the parent-child relationship. I constantly have to reiterate that I never wanted to hurt anyone, I only wanted to eat. I was gradually accepting that I would never know or attain social elegance, but alienation from my parents? I didn't expect that.

As days turned to weeks and weeks turned to months, middle school turned into nothing more than a collection of long-suffering memories. Semi-formal dances occurred where I was left unheld and social events occurred where I was left unnoticed. Society seemed to be fully content without my participation, rendering me a spectator in my own life. If it wasn't for my inconvenient circumference, I wonder how many people would have noticed me at all. I ate because I was unhappy and I was unhappy because I ate. To be honest, I felt less like a spectator and more like a prisoner.

As my middle school career was coming to an end, I reached such an apathetic state that my academic performance was falling apart as well. No longer were the ramifications of my actions contained to social and emotional endeavors. My grades became so poor that I was asked to leave the gifted program. "Asked to leave" is pleasant speak for "kicked out." Even my unshakable welcome in the world of hockey became suspect. My increasing girth made me noticeably slower than I used to be. I struggled just to keep up. While other sports are more accommodating to biggin' participation, hockey never quite picked up on the equal opportunity initiative.

Basketball welcomes thickness by placing such players in the middle of the paint and uses the player's size to "protect their house." For a point of reference, see Shaq, *not* Aaron Carter. Girth in football is a blessing, and in most cases, encouraged. There will always be a place for someone of size on the line as long as they can commit to picking up their block. However, in hockey, there is just is no place for it. When I was in possession of the puck, I had the ability to do things with it that kids twice my age couldn't do. It mattered very little because most of the time, I lacked the speed to even get to puck. Potential encased in failure; that seemed to be the ever-present story of my life. If there was an award for precision in blocking one's own shot, then at least I could claim one trophy.

My tale of mislay was finalized on the last day of amateur hockey tryouts. Centralized Pittsburgh Ice Hockey was not as much of a tradition around my school as a right of passage for anyone looking to take their on-ice performance to the next level. Anyone who was worth anything on their school team was also playing for Centralized.

Naturally, I convinced my parents that it was necessary for me to try out. After putting in what seemed like two days of ice hockey boot camp, I walked away from the tryouts feeling sore, confident, and accomplished. I put a few points on the board, I made a few key plays, and all in all, I felt pretty good.

Now, I'm not one to celebrate early, but making the team seemed like a lock. There were three options: Team AA, which were the elite of the elite; Team A, where the players had AA potential, but still needed some time to develop, and finally, there was Team B. The B team was where the leftovers ended up. I knew my inadequate agility would probably keep me out of the AA bracket, and I was okay with that. It was possible that I could make the A team, but I didn't really know any of the coaches. If for some reason I didn't make the A team, then my heart wouldn't be broken because at least I would play. This left me logically on the B team, a big fish on a small frozen pond, just how I liked it.

It made sense to me: not good enough to be elite, but still good enough to be on the team. So, I waited for my phone call and prepared my acceptance speech. A few days went by, I waited. Then a week went by, I waited some more. Two weeks went by and I was starting to get concerned. Finally, during a school hockey practice, Jordan was getting a hard time because he only made the A team. The laughing stopped, and all eyes turned to me as the question was asked:

So, what team did you make, Rochford?

Um, I'm not sure.
They haven't called me yet.

They haven't called you yet?
That's odd, practices start next week.
I'm sure they'll call you soon to let you know the news.

I put my head down to tie my skates while I acted like I didn't hear them laughing. I knew in my heart what news was forthcoming. When I got home, I sought out clarity by calling my team registration contact. Upon finally getting a live voice, I was thanked for my time as well as the hard work I put in. He informed me that all the roster spots had been assigned, but I was more than welcome to attend next year's tryouts. Somehow, the topic of refunding my deposit never came up. As the receiver turned from conversation to dial tone, the phone slowly fell from my hands onto the floor. I looked around the room as though I would find some sort of answer in all of this. Had I become so overweight that an organization would accept players of lesser ability rather than contend with the potential liability of my size? Why? It didn't make sense. They saw me score. They saw me drop the people who tried to hit me. It did not make sense. I kept looking around the room in hopes of finding an eleventh hour victory. Nothing came to mind except the dawning of a stress headache. As the room began to spin, I braced myself against the wall to catch my breath. Staring down at my shoes, a solitary tear fell. Failure had finally set in. I was defenseless against it. Lashing out, I began to yell at the wall.

B team! Are you serious? I couldn't even make the B team?!? Everyone who can show up on time and pay for registration makes the B team! They are the "participation award" of athletic team classification. Now you are telling me that I am too fat to even qualify for that?

U N B E L I E V A B L E!

I went over to the kitchen to drown my failure with a gallon of milk, a tub of crunchy peanut butter, and box of butter top crackers. I went downstairs and medicated until I felt the bloating overtake the sorrow. I awoke the next morning to the sound of my mother calling for me. As I struggled to get up, it was all that I could do to shake off the stench of dried dairy and self-loathing. I threw my tear-stained clothes from the night before towards the other side of the basement. Failing once again, my clothing hit door frame rather than making it through the opening. I walked over to pick them up and placed them in the hamper. Before I could do so, I stopped dead in my tracks. My attention became fixed upon the pile of ice hockey equipment that lay before me. I stared at it as though it was an unfaithful mistress who had broken every piece of my heart. I walked over to my skates in an attempt to rationalize the failure they had caused.

"All I wanted from you was enough speed to play for Centralized Pittsburgh just like everyone else. You couldn't even do that. You're dead to me!" I exclaimed as I threw my skates to the ground. Turning my back, I reprised by stating my current displeasure. "I just wanted to be social. I just wanted a reason to be able to have friends and eat. I guess that was too much to ask." It seems there is no way you can have your cake, and eat it too. Which, by-the-way, is the most ridiculous statement ever. What else is someone who is seeking out cake going to do with it other than eat it? This is by far the longest running, non-sensical statement, ever created. I mean, really? Really? Two thousand years later and this is as far as we've come? If for no other reason evolution is disproved by the longevity of this statement alone.

Further disproving progress was the fact that I was blaming inanimate equipment for my lack of ability. Those skates could only go as fast as I was able propel them, leaving my Bauer's fully pardoned of all wrongdoing. Hanging my head in further failure, I kicked my clothing over to the dirty laundry pile and headed for the shower. I used that opportunity to cry myself back to stability. I figured no one would hear the tears through the water.

After a few weeks of anti-social behavior, my mother suggested that I at least try to do something that would take my mind off of the situation. She encouraged me to take up a friend's offer to attend an all-night church event with his youth group. She believed it was just what I needed. "Who knows?" she said, "You just might have some fun and meet someone new, someone who will like you for what you can do, and not judge you for what you can't."

She was more than right. The first icebreaker of the evening was a 400-kid participation event in which I filled out a card with five pieces of information. The goal was to call out positive and obvious attributes until the last one standing won two tickets to a Pittsburgh Penguins game.

As the crowd dwindled from 400 to 25 kids, I realized that I was still standing. I also noticed a kid wearing a Montreal Canadiens hat. He looked like an actual hockey fan, and apparently I was staring too long, because our eyes were now making contact. He looked at me confused as I blurted out the only thing I knew about the Canadiens.

So, you're a Patrick Roy fan?

I spoke as though I had planned it all along.

Oh man, I love him,
you a Lemieux fan?

Nope, Ron Francis.

Huh, not my first choice,
but he's still pretty good.
I tell you what, if I win these tickets,
I'll take you.

You would do that?

Definitely.
You look like you would enjoy a game.

What's the catch?

Well, if you win, you have to take me.

That seems fair.

As contestants were picked off one by one, it came down to the two of us and three other kids. On the very next call, the announcer proclaimed:

"If you're wearing a hat of any sort, please sit down."

At first, we made eye contact. Then we looked at our respective hats. Looking back at each other, we sighed in unison, as we knew it was time to sit down. In the end, the hockey tickets wound up going to some blonde hottie who had no real concept of what she was even contesting for. However, it hardly seemed to matter. Once the tickets were awarded and we were dismissed from the mixer, I formally introduced myself to Montreal Canadiens Hat Kid. His name was Evan, and as it turned out, he was indeed a HUGE Patrick Roy fan.

As the night progressed, our conversation revealed Evan's desire to become the best goaltender he possibly could. This was great news and a fantastic opportunity for me. As you may remember, I was a spectacular goaltender who never got a chance to play forward. We put our heads together and contrived a plan to cultivate the finest of our abilities. I planned to teach him everything I knew about goaltending, and in return, I would use him as constant target practice to improve my offensive ability.

Looking beyond the hockey, it was nice to develop a stable friendship. For the next few months, Evan and I were inseparable. We played hockey all the time, and when we were not playing hockey, we were eating. When were done eating, we would play hockey some more. Our love for hockey was one of equal opportunity. Hockey playing, hockey card collecting and trading, watching hockey games and movies, partaking in hockey video games. We embraced it all.

It was so euphoric at times, I felt as though I was dreaming. For the first time in my life, I found contentment in something other than the seclusion of food. Evan had allowed me to be something that I never thought society would accept: myself.

Aside from hockey, it seemed as though Evan was teaching me valuable lessons in life as well. Such as how laughter can be used for social positioning. I never thought in a million years that my social awkwardness could be used for anything other than a reason to stifle my societal acceptance. But, there was Evan, using his rolls of chub to win over more laughs than insults. I'm not sure that I ever fully explained Evan's body type and personality; so allow me to do so. If you were to take the chubbiness and endearment of Oliver Hardy, John Candy, Chris Farley, Jack Black, and Seth Rogan, then proceed to divide it by five, you would have Evan. He somehow found that rarely attainable four-leaf clover of life, the harmonious coexistence of chubby and adorable.

Through observing him, I came to realize that every social group had their own lovable fat person. The trick is knowing what to look for. It could be that fun-loving uncle who eats far too much during the holidays, giving himself gas, which in turn ruins the night for the rest of us. It could be that big ol' lady you see at church every Sunday who just happens to be full of the Holy Ghost. She can't help herself from yelling AMEN as she encourages the preacher to "testify" at the conclusion of every single statement they make. It could even be that lovable grandmother who has to personally inspect every single portion she makes before it is free to leave her kitchen. How less rich would our lives be without these people? It seems to me that overweight people are like a good cup of coffee. Until you acquire their unique taste, you never fully appreciate them. Once you get acquainted with the combination of personality and flavor they have to offer, well, you couldn't imagine a day without them. As I navigated though a few of my own awkward situations, I tried to find the flavor of myself that would allow me to win over a few non-believers.

Through trial and error, I found that *Fat Guy Who Makes Fun of Himself* was the best option for me. Whether it was alluding to my multiple chins or my inability to fit into average sized clothing, I noticed that by making fun of me first, no one else would have the opportunity. After only a few short weeks of tweaking this mindset, I was able to transform my image from avoidably awkward fat kid into happy-go-lucky fat kid. Even though the term "fat kid" was still prevalent in descriptions, the ramifications of the term were not. For the first time in hormonal positioning, people no longer tried to avoid me. I wasn't awkward, I was just fat. I continued to use my intelligence to fend off insults. Once again, by thinking of better ways to insult myself than my adversaries, I was able to control this social war. It got to the point where bullies wouldn't even try because they knew their slams were insufficient to mine. It wasn't the ideal situation, but at least people were starting to accept me.

I took this newfound control and applied it to every situation possible. What came across as a jubilant attitude was actually a well-constructed plan to keep people laughing. If there is one thing observing Evan taught me, it was this: when people's hearts are filled with laughter, there is no room left in them for hate. Even if it was only temporary, I was through with being hated. I was well aware that they were laughing *at* me, and not *with* me. It did not matter, at least for the moment; they were laughing. Unfortunately, I had no idea that this emotional stimulus would lead to a deficit of epic proportions. One in which teenage Jeremy would be forced to pay at the hands of crippling emotional weakness for years to come.

Chapter 7:

Love Is a Verb; But What Is Alienation?

!!!!!!!!!!!PPPPPPPPPPIIIIIIIIIINNNNNNNNNNGGGGGGGGGG!!!!!!!!!!!!

Oh man...Did you see that?

JEREMY!!!! NOW IS NOT THE TIME!!!!

Yeah, I know. But did you see that?
They almost took Jeff's head off!

Dude, Seriously! Pay attention or you're next!

I thought gym class was supposed to be fun!
I don't think I like this!

I know, but I don't think that you have a choice.

Well that's hardly fair. This is ninth grade,
we're almost adults...Rich....LOOK OUT!!!!

!!!!!!!!!!!PPPPPPPPPPIIIIIIIIIINNNNNNNNNNGGGGGGGGGG!!!!!!!!!!!!

Johnson, you've been hit. Sit down.

Oh man. What do I do now?
This turning into such a cliché!

Who are you talking to now?
Everyone from your team
is sitting on the bleachers.

I know. I am having an internal
monologue moment.

Is that sane?
I mean, do people still do that?

Yes, of course it is.
This is how the normal hide their
innormality from the rest of the world.
It happens all the time.

Look out!!!

Wait, what?

!!!!!!!!!!!PPPPPPPPPPIIIIIIIIIINNNNNNNNNNGGGGGGGGG!!!!!!!!!!!

OH COME ON!
In the face? Really? Ugh!
Oh no, did I just wet myself?

No, that's just sweat.
Remember, you are quite portly.
Other than that, you have a
facial contusion and a bruised ego.

Thank you "self,"
where were you a minute ago?

Hey I said, "Look out"!
You were too busy trying to
justify that an internal
monologue was normal.

!!!!!!!!!!!!!!!!!!!!!ROCHFORD...YOU'RE OUT...!!!!!!!!!!!!!!!!!!!!!
ALL RIGHT MEN, SHOWER UP!!

You know, I'm not sure I can
handle four more years of this.

Yeah, it doesn't look positive.

Again, thanks. Do you think in the future you will
be able to give me better guidance and possibly
not freeze up in high-pressure situations?

Yeah. Um...that's not looking too good, either.
Actually, you probably shouldn't
count on me for too much at all.
Don't forget, I am still a part of your subconscious.
I am only as good as you make me.

Swell.

With the grace of a phoenix and the sting of a dodge
ball, my high school career had officially begun.

So whatever became of that shower?

What? Really? Thanks... I was hoping the readers would have forgotten about that. I already snuck by without telling them about my fear of moobage.

Moobage?

Yes, moobage. Being as large as I was, I had very little control over where the fat chose to accumulate throughout my body. Basic physical law suggests that there are only so many places it could possibly settle. Let me just say by the tender age of 14, I was more endowed than most college girls. Meaning I had man boobs, or moobs.

Wait. What? Huh?

Yeah. And truthfully, I don't feel comfortable speaking about them. Or putting myself in situations where I have to share my moobs with people.

Whoa man. That is way too much information.
Clearly you have thought about this way too much.
I am assuming you have encountered
situations like this before?

Yes, sir. Middle school aquatic physical education. Needless to say, that one took a little bit of creativity. I, being a male, did not have quite the same equipment that the ladies do. This left me with fewer options in terms of excuses. However, I did retain a few grown-up friends from back in my baseball card days. I simply convinced them to write a few notes stating that I

was allergic to chlorine, and therefore, unable to participate in
any pool-based activities.

How exactly did you convince them?

Money, of course.
And a few baseball cards here and there.

And that worked?
I mean, the teachers just bought it?

Without question. They had to.

They had to?

Yeah, everyone was afraid of being
politically incorrect. The public
school system was no different.

I see. But I thought you weren't going to lie anymore.

Yeah, I thought so, too. But, when it came down to it,
I felt worse from the way I was treated over my girth than
I felt from the conviction of lying. I just don't think people
realize the amount of fear that the overweight person lives in.
The fear of rejection. The fear of hate. Even worse, the fear
that every derogatory remark made just might be accurate.

I see. Wow, man, that's heavy. No pun intended.
Wait, wait; that may have saved you from the pool,
but the water used for showering is treated
in a completely different manner.

Well, middle school was pretty easy. There was no need to shower since no swimming had actually occurred. However, high school was a completely different story. I reached a point in my academic tenure where I could no longer avoid showering in group situations. Though no swimming had occurred, enough sweat was perspired to warrant a cleansing. Before this point gets lost, I need you to remember that 99.9% of my actions were designed to maintain as much dignity as possible.

It is with this in mind I propose showering topless with men was much more dignified at that point than wearing a chub-concealing tank top while swimming with females. The rationale being this: guys in a locker room situation make fun of you no matter what. If your body is blessed, you get made fun of. If your body is lacking, you get made fun of. Everyone is a little too fat, a little too gay, a little too hairy, a little too hairless. By taking off my shirt in front of them, I placed the option of ridicule in their hands. But, if they chose to comment on my manly northern blessings, then I had every right to question their sexual preferences for noticing them.

Well played, sir. Go on.

Fate, further proving it is still no fan of mine, decided to schedule my gym class in the middle of the day. This meant that I had to shower. It is one thing to be known as the fat kid, it's an entirely different level to be known as the SMELLY fat kid. So, there I was, ready to place my theorem into action. To reduce the amount of eyes that could possibly fall upon me, I began doing remedial tasks until the locker room had mostly cleared. I piddled around with my shoelaces, unfolded and refolded clothing, organized my travel bathroom kit. Whatever tactics I could use to look busy, I did. Once I felt it was clear enough, I darted into the shower, turning on all of the water and rinsed off as quickly as I possibly could. NO SMELLY FAT KIDS HERE, I mentally proclaimed!

While my wait and conquer approach operated flawlessly, it didn't mean the plan itself was perfect. By the time I actually got into the shower, all of the warm water was used from everyone else who showered before me. Needless to say, my in-school showering method lacked enjoy-ability in every sense of the word. Arctic sensation aside, what bothered me most about the cold water was its ability to awaken my sensitive moobage to a level of perk that was far beyond necessary.

In an attempt to make the process somewhat tolerable, I began to practice my wait and conquer approach during my morning shower routine. My goal was to desensitize my moobs to the point that water temperature was no longer an issue. This plan also failed, as I merely gained a useless superpower of cutting glass. Adding insult to injury, it made me hate waking up in the morning more than ever. It's one thing to face a relentless school day of ridicule, it's another to do it while mammarically saluting. I do admit, while I am largely responsible for this shower debacle. I also hold the towel industry partially at fault.

What?

Up until then, average bath towels would wrap completely around me. But had become so large that those *one size fits all* towels no longer covered **all** of me. Their standard cloth

91

dimensions could not wrap around my waist. I guess I was a part of the reason why one size fits all had to be amended. Once I graduated to beach-towel living in everyday situations, another adventure had begun. Where in the world would I find an acceptable beach towel during non-swimming seasons? Nothing is ever simple when you are overweight. Life just isn't designed for plus sized living. Do you have any further questions?

No. I'm good. As you were.

Thanks.

With all of those considerations aside, my high school introduction had not gone as badly as it could have. At least I told myself that until I believed it. I figured it like this: no one really fits in during their first week. Everybody is a new face and the imperfections we bring are fair game for whoever wants to love them or hate them accordingly.

With that being said, I would also be lying if I did not mention all the fail-safe's most freshmen have upon entry. Junior varsity athletes became varsity athletes. Prep band members became marching band members. Pre-algebra clubbers became mathletes. The socially unaware remained socially unaware, showing off their high fives and finger snaps to everyone who hated them for it.

But what becomes of the rest of us? I was too large to be imaginary. I couldn't just be rounded off. Where do the remainders fit in? Student council, perhaps? Nope, I failed at running my own life well, I couldn't imagine leading others. By applicable association, this also eliminated the mock trial team, Key Club, and Rotary Club. My inability to sing combined with my lack of metronomic prowess eliminated jazz and concert band. I had lost visual contact with my feet. If there is one thing history has taught us, it is that syncopating anything with phantoms is completely impossible. Good day to you, marching band. My not-so-honorable discharge from advanced academics and my dismissal from the honors program lead to a blacklisting from the journalism and mathletic clubs. I could barely grasp the native language of my own homeland, so naturally, I was embargoed from the French and Spanish clubs.

Within the confines of my own mind I was hopelessly awkward. It elevated when I was aware people were paying attention to me. Drama club, please exit stage left. I had to wonder what was left to embrace aside from a nomadic lifestyle of wandering the hallways of social ostracism. I really hoped there was more to the rest of my life than merely trying to survive.

Being proactive, I lobbied myself to any remaining social group that would allow me to join. Time and time again, I found that my inability to contribute anything made them all thoroughly unaccepting. In the wake of treading social water, I found my friends moving on to forge their own identities. Some of them realized their untapped athletic ability and found team-based acceptance. Others concluded they weren't nearly as dumb as they were lazy and set their sights on higher education. Some discovered their voice both figuratively and literally through the performing arts. Evan, well, he took his fat and funny act to a level that left mine far behind.

As for me, I found myself walking home alone, once again trying to hold back whatever tears I could. I longed for the desirable touch of social interaction, but continued to settle for the taste of salty and sweet. It's not that I didn't enjoy life; I just wasn't any good at it. My parents continually encouraged me to look beyond social barriers. They knew how emotionally unhealthy I was becoming. I would overhear them voicing their concerns on a daily basis. "He used to be so social and outgoing. I wonder what happened to him," they would whisper. The hardest part to convey to anyone was that nothing really happened to me. Other than a couple of extra pounds, I was still the same person I was in middle school. I just came to terms with the fact that society does not embrace fat people.

Life just isn't designed for those who excel in abdominal expansion. Seat belts became more constrictive than beneficial. I felt more at ease using my 50 plus-inch traveling airbag than I did being suffocated by belted nylon. My inability to maneuver inside of a restaurant was dismal. I was just about to outgrow booth seating. Even going to the bathroom was becoming a foreign task. If the door swung outward then that was fine, it was just a question of landing gear alignment. However, if the door opened inward, well, let's just say it became a brilliant dance that was nothing close to gazelle-like.

The media never helped. Commercials forced me to self-loathe in the hopes that I would purchase a weight-loss solution. Trying to find comfort in Hollywood was as useless then as it is now. From The Breakfast Club to American Pie to Napoleon Dynamite, they all seem to cover the angst of growing up from every social and emotional perspective, except one. Obesity. We are impossible to miss, and always overlooked. It seems as though the media can only portray the overweight as slobs who lack all self-control and social ambition. Unless eating is involved, then there is a desire to be proficient. But wait. Not all hope is lost. Lest we forget what follows any successful mealtime consumption. Think about any fat role you have seen. What is it? The need to expel waste! It is the one and only thing the obese are able to excel at! And Hollywood embraces all forms. Liquids, solids, and gas all seem to pass through the canals of the obese as just quickly and awkwardly as they were consumed. It's sad.

The fat *guy* never gets the girl. The fat *girl* never seems to be the love interest unless it is part of some malicious prank. There is just no valor in overweight living. I cannot tell you how insulted I am every time I watch a television personality step into a fat suit to emulate what it must feel like. This must-see television is no social experiment, it was my day-to-day existence. This was my life and all they did was laugh at it. There was no camera that stopped rolling. There were no second or third takes. My sub-conscious was my only audience, and it never shut off. Only when my head hit the pillow was I finally free enough to embark on the nocturnal romancing of a life where weight was no longer a social factor. Back to an easier time, before hormones and social positioning eliminated the innocence of childhood.

I can still remember going to the park and not having a care in the world. I would play in the sandbox and become friends with anyone who wanted to help me build the biggest sand castle ever. But then life got in the way, and everything changed. When I found myself in public, people unnecessarily kept their distance. They saw me coming and avoided me as though obesity was some form of contractible airborne disease. While at the park, I understood my weight eliminated seesaw from my range of recreation.

It wasn't just the park, it was the mall, it was the bus,

and it was anywhere public interaction occurred. I could not avoid being avoided. I really wonder what everyone was so afraid of. What amazes me most was that in a world that desired nothing more than change, we have allowed intolerance to become absolutely tolerable. A great comedian once joked,

"Plastic surgery is a fantastic invention because it allows the outside of oneself to accurately reflect the inside. Fake."

A society based on character, not glamour. Now that would be change I could believe in.

Chapter 8:

Waisting Away

Whoever spoke the words, "Tis better to have loved and lost than to have never have loved at all," must have never been overweight. The poetry of the statement offers such a great amount of false hope. Well, at least that's how I perceived it. Maybe some people can treat a kind, loving relationship as though it was commonplace; but I never had that good fortune. When someone is as large as I was, the opportunity for finding love or even an occasional snuggle is almost non-existent.

Before we proceed, I feel that I must confess something to you. Come here. A little closer. Great. My dirty little secret to all of you is how little food mattered to me at this point of the story. I know I have made a big deal about eating and that is what I want to focus on for a brief moment. Very seldom was it the taste of food that attracted me to it. Don't get me wrong, I consumed many delicious items; but more important than the taste was the euphoria I felt as I went through the eating process. The aroma of the food as it passed under my nose and into my mouth. The chess game of biting, chewing, tasting, swallowing and breathing. Food was merely the tool that allowed me to escape, if only for a moment, from all of my inequities. I could have just as easily chosen drugs, alcohol, or cutting, but I didn't. Mayonnaise captured my heart, and per kilo, it had a much cheaper street value.

Joking aside, there was nothing that propelled me to

eat more than the feeling of unbridled emotional acceptance I received from it. I imagine the thrill of one's first kiss was the same flutter my heart felt during the moments of consumption. But at that point, I had never kissed a girl, so how would I know?

Shamefully, my condition only drew female attention for the purposes of entertainment and protection. No one cared about the person I was or someday hoped to become. People only spoke to me when they needed something from me or if I was inconveniently in their way. The only constant I had in my life were the waiting arms of the food I had yet to consume. How was it that I was completely surrounded by society and at the exact same time, so completely alone? It was as though I had been cast away to the three-island cluster off of the coast of "Everyoneishappyexceptforyouland." Allow me to be your tour guide through this purgatorial side trip.

The first island we come across is the most isolated of the three. Our limited findings suggest that most natives to Island 1 are forsaken romantics. While this island is impossible to miss, it's amazing that society has found it just as impossible to notice. The climate is fairly lethargic and non-indigenous to romance. This has allowed researchers to establish broken hearts and tear stains as Island 1's primary export. While the island is co-ed, the inhabitants rarely attempt to circumvent their circumstances through each other. This baffles researchers because the very characteristics that bind inhabitants to this island might just be the very same characteristics that would allow them to leave.

The second island, located in the near distance, is a quaint little commonwealth known as "Friendzoneopia."

Friends and acquaintances of Island 1 are the main inhabitants of this quandarafiable region. The strictly platonic interaction between Island 1 and Island 2 has astounded researchers for years. While occupants are remarkably compatible and their companionship would balance out each other's inequities, the inhabitants of Island 2 never desire anything more than sustainable friendship with the inhabitants of Island 1. Even more perplexing to researchers is how remarkably one-sided the communication is. Transmissions from Island 2 flow directly to Island 1 with 3- to 5G-network clarity. Every time Island 2 beckons Island 1 concerning their current relational status, it is received clearly and static-free. The true phenomenon is observed by Island 2's inability to process relevant verbalization from Island 1. Even though communication is designed to flow both ways, it never quite occurs. This means that all of the great advice given from Island 1 never makes it to the ears of Friendzoneopia. The ability of Island 2's inhabitants to painfully make the same mistakes over and over and over again has proven our researchers' communication plight as more than just theory.

The third island that finalizes our geographical displacement is the nation of "Outofyourleaguedreamlover." This landmass is unique due to its ever-changing incumbents, as well as Island 1's perception of them. While visual observation from Island 1 to Island 3 is impeccably clear, the same cannot be said for the contrary. Likewise, verbal association between Island 3 and Island 1 is just as non-substantial. Due to lack of communication between the two islands, as well as Island 3's inability to recognize Island 1's existence, many researchers believe Island 3 may actually be a mirage derived from an over-exaggerated fantasy thriving off of Island 1's under-stimulation.

However, researchers who were able to examine and experience the emotional process of an Island 1 native unequivocally discern that their pain and overwhelming void is far too authentic to be fabricated.

Jeremy! JEREMY ROCHFORD!
Are you sleeping in class again?

No? Wait, what? No! I'm not sleeping in class!

Okay then, Mr. Rochford, what is X equivalent to?

Wait. What?

You heard me. I just got done explaining
to the class what Y and R are equal to.
If you were paying attention, i.e.,
NOT SLEEPING, then you will have no
problem telling the class what X is equivalent to.

Um....I...ah....

You have no idea, do you, Mr. Rochford?

No, ma'am.

Yeah, didn't think so. Go to the office and
tell them why I sent you.

Yes, ma'am...

As Jeremy sheepishly exits the classroom, a familiar voice accompanies him down the long corridor to the principal's office.

So what are you going to tell them?

Oh hey, it's you. How nice of you to join us.
Fantastic job back there with that whole
math debacle thing.
I could have actually used you.

Man, we have been over this.
I am a being of your subconscious.
Therefore, I am only as useful as
you are willing to make me.

I hate you. I hate you so much.

All pleasantries aside,
you do have a situation at hand.

I know. I'm aware.

And while my obnoxiously faltering subconscious was correct, it did very little to prevent or address the fact that in that moment, I was on my way to the principal's office to attempt to explain my class-time slumber. It is at this very moment, I must press pause on this flashback to tell you a background story.

My father loves computers. He loves the way they work, the way they save him time, the way they streamline his existence, and most importantly, the way they make him a very efficient individual. You can say that I lived in a very technologically blessed household. His desire to instill a similar love for computers in both my sister and I started at an early age with an Apple IIGS. This computer was purchased to help with math homework and to sharpen our word processing abilities. My sister used it for those reasons, but I decided to turn it into countless nights of Oregon Train and California Games. I couldn't footbag to save my life, but I was amazing at avoiding dysentery.

However, it wasn't 1848, it was 1996. The internet was just becoming a household option, and my father made sure that we were well equipped. Like most things in my life, I found a way to abuse it. I figured if this *could* be used for accessing a world of knowledge, what could it possibly do for electronic social networking? I'm not going to lie to you; engaging in human interaction with individuals who cared about my thoughts was amazing, whether it was electronic or otherwise. It was just so much more rewarding than a fake connection with those who really felt I was not worth their time in a non-digital reality.

The online lifestyle was fantastic for me. It gave me the freedom to be myself or create whatever reality I wanted to. I even took the time to manufacture an adorable little Jeremy avatar (Which turned into an even cuter "Mii" ten years later). I mean look at cyber me, he's so adorable. Why wouldn't you want to electronically flirt with that sexy redhead? He is the pot of gold at the end of the rainbow.

Anyways, like all of my other schemes, this one started out slowly with no real intention of manipulation. I say that because I honestly believed that. I never manufactured these ideas with the belief that someone would actually get hurt. Or furthermore, that I might actually get caught. I think my brain lacked the filter that should catch bad ideas and send them back for cerebral review until they become refined into a good idea. Even to this day I still think I lack that filter. Like one of my favorite comedians, my mind works more like a baseball game without an on-deck circle. Straight from the bench to the plate and then it's batter up!

With that reckless mentality, I nightly adorned my computer with multiple scholastically-themed browsers as well as a word processor for the appearance of greater academia. While all of that occurred on the surface, I maintained a silently minimized version of AIM beneath for conversational pleasure. When my parents passed through, they saw me working diligently to move my education forward all the while I was really studying how to become a cyber stud. Those social deviations started as a weekly occasion, but the more successful I became, the more time I invested.

I fell in love with this social life I never thought I could obtain. My parents were none the wiser. To keep them from asking too many questions, I stayed diligent with my academic angle until they retired upstairs for the evening. Once I knew they were asleep (no movement with snoring was my cue), I was free to partake in every chat room that I could find. ICQ, CompuServe, Prodigy, and AOL were all at my fingertips.

Before I knew it, my weekly social wander had turned into a nightly marathon. And those nightly marathons were about to catch up to me...
right...
about...
now.

In hopes of stalling the inevitable, I walked as slowly as I possibly could. I had no idea what I was going to tell my principal. See, this is where a good schemer has a contingency plan. I wish I had that filter. I wanted to use something that had to do with being sick. Administrative folk normally eat that kind of stuff up. I knew how to fake a headache pretty well. But I actually fell asleep, so I couldn't use the "I didn't fall asleep, I merely put my head down" excuse. I guess I could have, but I never brought it up at the point of accusation. That oversight left me seriously overwhelmed if it were to come down to a teacher vs. student truth-off. With that option eliminated, what else could have kept me up all night that was not only fakeable, but also untraceably feasible? Observe.

"Mrs. Igloo, I am so sorry for falling asleep today in math class. I did so with no disrespect to Mrs. Isosceles. You see, I was up all night with an awkward stomach pain, a headache, and other sickness-related things that I am sure you really don't want to hear about. Bottom line is I have a group video project due and I am the only one with the editing ability. If it were a situation where I was the only one depending on me, then I guarantee you I would have stayed home. But, my entire group is depending on me advancing this project and I am just not the kind of guy who likes to let people down. So, I came to school anyway. I feel my falling asleep in class is a by-product of my insufficient slumber, over-the-counter medication, and trying to maintain the balance of keeping down what was going in, and a waning interest in polynomials."

Indeed, this defense worked out just fine. I walked into the office and after approximately fifteen minutes of playing my role, I was off to the school nurse to obtain my mandatory note of medical clearance. It wasn't so much to send me home, as it was to ensure my condition was curable with an aspirin or two. After receiving an a-okay, I sat there until the bell rang. Once it did, I lethargically merged into pedestrian traffic to rejoin my daily activities. I walked towards the lunchroom (I wanted I to catch a preview of my afternoon delight options). Try as I might to concentrate on Mexican pizza Wednesday, my attention was drawn to the fragrance of Bath& Figure works permeating in front of me. Who could it be, none other than Mary Ann.

As a personal rule, I tried to minimize any attraction I could possibly have towards anyone. Don't get me wrong; I think females are God's greatest creation. Sadly though, I found that having a crush on a girl is like being an orphan at Christmas. Why long for something so far out of reach? It just seems cruel.

Yet, somehow, there was always something that kept my eyes wandering to Mary Ann. She was a prefect blend of cute and sassy. During the warm months, she wore adorable little sundresses that made my heart melt. Beyond that, she was a member of the honors program and played a secondary role in the drama club. Problem being, other than mostly everything about me, Mary Ann was in the exact same math class that I consistently fell asleep in. With her high standards and my sagging waistline, there was no way she would fall for someone like me.

Fairytales happen with kissable frogs, not bloated manatees. I wonder how many other hearts are beating out of rhythm with me at this very moment.

Chapter 9:

The Onion Ring of Dante's Inferno

There was a time in my life when back-to-school shopping genuinely excited me. The smell of a brand new Trapper Keeper mixed with a crisp new backpack was enough to make me lose sleep for days. What kind of pencils would I get? I was never sure, but I always thought they were AWESOME!

However, once high school happened, everything changed. What was an enjoyable shopping experience became a silent war of social positioning. Defining ones style and choosing name brand logos became as important as looking both ways before crossing the street. It was tolerable for a while because most stores had a "BIG" man's section with some fashionable items.

My junior year, however, I reached the end of the line. What should have been a great day of bargain hunting deteriorated into nothing more than an exercise in futility. My mother and I hit store after store in an attempt to replenish my food-stained wardrobe. As we did, we consistently came up empty-handed. We could find nothing respectable that would fit me. We were completely at a loss for words. We were so aggravatingly lost that we didn't know what to do...so...we decided to quit for the day.

On the drive home, the silence became so awkward that it was deafening. After her fourth cigarette in about five minutes, my mother finally lost it.

What's next, Jeremy? Where does this end?
You are a 16-year-old kid and we can't even
find clothes that fit you in the husky sections of stores.
The only options you have are button down shirts
that make you look like a clown, racing t-shirts,
or apparel that a biker would wear!
I mean, where do we go from here?
Do you think the Big & Tall has
normal clothing that would fit you? I don't know.
I've never shopped at a Big & Tall.
Would they have things you could wear?

How would I know?
I've never shopped there either.

Needless to say, this was not how I envisioned life as a 16-year-old. When we arrived home, I ran through the door and headed straight to my bedroom. My mother didn't send me there, nor was she punishing me for this situation, I just needed some time to be alone. I needed time to think. I needed to clear my mind. I needed to eat. As I sat there looking at the package of half-consumed Double Fills cookies, I couldn't help but hear the echoes of my mother's outburst.

Where does this stop?

I mean really, where does it? How does this end? I couldn't answer that because I had no idea. I mean, it would eventually end when I die, but I never wanted it to come to that. I never thought it would.

I wanted nothing more than to lose weight, but I had no idea where to begin. Being supportive isn't yelling at someone until they hate themselves, and my issues were far beyond anything a diet cola could fix. Everyone told me that all I needed to do was just eat less. For people like me, it wasn't that simple. Food was the only comfort I had in my life. So, I was stuck there having to choose between my happiness or my health. I shouldn't have to make that choice, I was too young.

I walked over to my closet. I opened the door and gazed upon the rails of clothing that no longer fit me. I thought to myself, "Where did we go wrong guys, where did we all go wrong? How long has it been since anything actually fit me? How long has it been since I wore any of this? Why do I even keep this closet full?" My clothing was nothing more than a reminder of a poorly lived life.

I slammed the closet door and nearly ran into the dresser. It felt like the room was getting smaller and smaller. Or, maybe I just kept getting larger and larger. I opened each drawer in the hopes of finding something I forgot about that would be size-appropriate. Like the rest of my life, I found nothing except unwanted mockery. My daily serving of it was brought forth by mounds and mounds of sweatpants and underwear. All of which had elastic that was stretched out far beyond the point usefulness. So far in fact, they had become broken. I mean really, how fat do you have to be to break a pair of sweatpants?

How symbolic of the way I felt, broken and useless. I wondered if my underwear hated its existence as much as I hated mine. I guess it could have been worse; we both could have been toilet seats. I wouldn't wish the life of a toilet seat upon anyone. Honestly, I don't think I would have wished my life at that point upon anyone, either. I just wished I was normal. I wished I could wear clothing that made me feel good about myself rather than paranoid. I wished I didn't have to fight with a mirror every time I walked by one. I just wished I could have looked forward to facing the day for once in my life.

I grew tired of conversing with myself as I wiped the tears away from my eyes. In doing so, I concluded that I needed to be anywhere but there. I told my parents I was going ice skating as I left the house to seek clarity and closure once again. But I wasn't going ice skating, I was heading out to find a solution. My mother may have been too proud to shop in Big & Tall clothing stores, but I had surrendered my dignity a long time ago.

I passed by the bank and withdrew a quick $100 on way to the gas station to fill up my van. Noticing a sandwich shop in this convenient location, I decided that a mutual fill-up would be necessary. As my eyes wandered, I found the statement, "Eat all you want and still lose weight. No exercise required!" captivated my very soul. It spoke to me like angels singing in unison. This had to be too good to be true. Eat all you want and still lose weight with out any exercise? I thought that it must have been designed specifically for me because I not only wanted to lose weight, but I wanted to do it without exercise. I read further. "Get rid of body fat without leaving your house."

What? Yes! Sign me up!

My attention was captured by these pill-sized messiahs. In a moment of weakness, I purchased two bottles with my meal. Now how did they work? Let's read. Take four pills before each meal for best results. This must have been for *normal* cases of weight loss. I believed that I fell into the extreme category, so I thought I would take eight. I wondered if there was a warning about overdosing...nope. The only warning stated, "These claims have not been proven by the FDA" and "Results are not typical."

Wait, "Results not typical?" What a downer. I mean, these pills had to work, right? Companies can't just print whatever they want to in order to sell a product. That would be very manipulative to my already vulnerable state as a consumer and as an individual.

With all of the excitement I had almost forgotten about the task at hand. I polished off my sandwich, jumped in the car, and headed back to the store where my mother and I were shopping earlier. Making my way back through the husky section, I couldn't help but notice those 3XL t-shirts with the utility pocket looked a lot better the second time around (knowing now that they were my only option). I also noticed a few racing t-shirts which only helped to prove my mother right. I had no idea who any of the drivers were, but for the next few months I had no choice but to be their biggest fan.

Since it was close to closing time, I found myself with umpteen other individuals waiting in line for the **ONE** cashier that was open in the entire store. There was a really attractive girl in front of me, but unfortunately she was with a really mean-looking boyfriend. You know the type, those guys who look like they should be the drummer for an unnecessarily aggressive rock band. Yeah, he was that guy. So I couldn't make any kind of visual contact with those people. Behind me was a big old lady who smelled like cats and hamburgers. Hmm.

I wished I wasn't so awkward. I wished I didn't have an inner monologue. Do other people talk to themselves? I wondered if I had enough money for all of those shirts. Yeah, I was fine. Until I noticed that all of the racing shirts had an alcohol or tobacco sponsor written all over them. I couldn't wear those to school. I'd seen students get in trouble over their Master P "No Limit Soldier" t-shirts because they might have advocated gang violence. I could have only imagined the stories I would have had to make up to pull off those shirts.

I HATED MY LIFE. It never got easier. Why couldn't I have good attributes? I paid for my shirts and as I was walking out the door, a group of scantily clad drunk girls stumbled through, with one of them literally running into me. As she latched onto my shoulder to keep from falling over, her friend grabbed her just as quickly and said "Ew Kourtney, you definitely don't want that one, he's a fatty."

What was that all about?

I have no idea.

Had you not been there,
that girl would have absolutely bit it.

I'm aware.

So....you save her and you still get made fun of

Yep.

There comes a time when you really have to question if there is a God at all. How could a loving God really let something that embarrassing happen to someone so downtrodden? That is another book, for another time...

I had to get home for some shirt customization. No, I was not going to bedazzle around the sexy pocket of my plain t-shirts, rather, I was merely going to stretch them out to ensure they didn't bunch up and cling to me in all of those "man places". To some of you, this happens all of the time. To others, you have no idea what I am talking about because you just throw on a shirt and don't have to think twice.

For those of you who may not know the process, allow me to explain. First, you sit securely on the corner of the bed. Second, you bend your knees with your feet perched on the corner of the bed. Once you are stable, pull the bottom of the shirt securely over your knees and stretch it as far as you possibly can. Not only does this make the shirt 10 times more comfortable, it also makes an adorable bell-shaped hang. I call it the reverse umbrella. Comfort aside, it was my way of fighting back at the fabric that was slowly suffocating my will to live. I admit, this was not the most dignifying thing in the world to do, but it sure beat looking like a sausage day in and day out.

I put away my purchases, took off my t-shirt and stood in front of the mirror. What was it about my body that made people hate me? The echoes of my mother and Kourtney still rang in my head. Regardless of how it looked or how it made them feel, I was still a human being.

All that stress perpetuated a massive headache in me that could not be ignored. It needed to be dealt with it in a way that would take my mind off of everything that occurred. I called Evan to see if he wanted to shoot some hockey. He couldn't, he was busy. I called another friend to see if he wanted to go to the mall; he had a date. I wished I had a date. I called a few others; they too were all busy.

Forget it; I thought to myself. I couldn't stay there. Those walls were suffocating me. I put my shirt back on, reached for my keys, and headed out to drive the town once more. I rode around for hours screaming at the top of my lungs along with the music, all the while confessing my greatest fears and failures to any part of the dashboard that would listen.

If I was so good at convincing everyone that I was happy being the fat guy, why couldn't I convince those same people to like me? All I wanted right then was to fall into someone's arms and have them tell me everything would be okay. But it never would be okay, would it? I was never going to be okay! AND I STILL HAD A HEADACHE! I was done.

I made the next left turn which took me into the drive-thru of Captain Tasty's Fish & More Emporium. I always found comfort and clarity in their 5-piece bonanza meal. Three pieces of fish, two pieces of chicken, french fries, coleslaw, two hush puppies, and an extra large Dr. Zepper always gave me a rarely attainable peace. For those extra contemplative and lengthy nights, I added an additional ten hush puppies and twenty packets of tartar sauce for extra clarity.

With my food in hand and my heart on my sleeve, I drove to the highest level of Adventure World's parking lot for a little contemplative stargazing. "Are people like me ever meant to be happy?" I thought to myself. I mean, singularly I could handle the lack of female interest, the unnecessary fat kid comments, the consistent personal disappointment, the awkwardness of clothes, the unease of social situations, and the lethargical-ness that caused me to fall asleep in class. On a good day, I could even rationalize the constant letdown that I was to my parents. All I seemed to do was drain their wallets and patience.

But it was that perfect storm effect I found to be

overwhelming. I just didn't understand why all of this had to happen to me. I think what bothered me more was that whiny skinny people complained about the most petty of issues. I mean, how sad was my existence that their problems would have been a reprieve from my everyday life? *I* had to choose which restaurants I ate at based not upon the type of food they served, but rather, if their booth would be large enough to accommodate me. I had to lift, tuck, wiggle, and hold my breath in order to fit myself into one of our school's all-in-one desk/chair combos. It took not one, not two, but three, at least three stress-filled, deliberate presses to secure my seatbelt.

They on the other hand, were worried about who they were going to take to homecoming because three girls asked them, but only one could be selected. Even worse, they had the audacity to plan on dismissing the other two in a way that left their options open in case the one they did choose would not live up to expectations. Do you know how it felt to go to the movies and see people like that with a girl on their arm, shamelessly showing their exploratory PDA without giving it a second thought?

"I mean God, how is this fair? My only affection comes from a large popcorn with malted milk balls. How do these people get to live in sinful debauchery and I get punished for it? More importantly, why don't you ever answer me? I wish you would answer my prayers. You know what, it really doesn't matter. I clearly do not figure into your omnipotent plans for my happiness. I'm over it." I thought out loud.

By this time it had gotten rather late and I figured it was best I head home; I was sure my earthly father was getting concerned about my whereabouts. Contemplating the harsh words I had for the God I was starting to doubt made for a pensive drive home. As I walked in the door, my parents were watching TV in the living room to stay awake. They wanted to make sure I made it home safely. After a bit of small talk, I headed up the stairs and back into my bedroom. I walked in, kicked off my shoes, and hit the lights. I sat by the window and gazed upon the same stars as before. I wondered if anyone out there was looking at the same stars and feeling just as lost as I was. I couldn't hold back my tears any longer, so I decided I should just let out a good cry.

My tears slowly turned into snores, snores turned into dreams, and before I knew it, the night turned into dawn. While eating breakfast, I decided to break the ice: "Mom, there is no need for us to go clothes shopping today. I found a bunch of clothing at the bottom of my drawers last night that I had forgotten about. They will do just fine for right now." She looked at me half awake and half confused as she responded with an obligatory sigh. I knew she was in no mood for fighting when she said, "If that's what makes you happy." It was.

I grabbed my toasty-tarts and headed for the door. "Hey Mom, I'm going to the driving range to get some exercise." "Be safe," she replied. With a heart full of questions and a CD player full of Green Day, I jumped in the van and hit the road. Once again, I was not going to the driving range. It had actually been closed for years, but my mother didn't know those things. No, I was headed to the exact same field I found myself at the night before with even more questions and less hope. I wasn't sure what I hoped to find by going there and talking to the morning sky, but it never stopped me from going. As I settled on a park bench, I began to lose myself in the calming nature of the wind-pushed clouds.

I have to admit, watching those clouds frolic like they had no care in the world made me a little bit jealous. They were free to float away from any stormy weather while I was stuck there, condemned to carry the weight of social politics on my shoulders and the weight of myself on my poor back. I didn't think I would ever understand why evolution had failed me. I turned my head to see a fly struggling in a spider's web and I felt like at least something knew how I felt. Poor little guy. I wondered if he knew that in the wild, only the strong survive. It's just unfortunate that some creatures have a more graceful defense than others.

Let's use the turtle and the snail, for example. These species in no way have the ability to oppose or even to outrun most of their natural predators. However, nature has given them an ideal defense mechanism. Both are equipped with a hardened shell to retreat into and wait out whatever attack is forthcoming. By doing so, the snail and turtle have an opportunity to live another day.

I, on the other hand, seemed to have no refuge from my predators at all. Maybe that's the point I was missing. Maybe that mini-breakdown was supposed to be a great metaphor. Maybe I was supposed to view high school as nature's attack on me. Maybe my "shell" was the armor of my creative wit, which I should have used to deflect hateful words and the negative glares of my surroundings. On paper it sounded all well and good, but I was in no mood to deal with two more years of retreating.

That seems like an overly elaborate explanation to prove such a minor point. My issues were not directly affecting others. The choice to super size myself did not directly cause a child to starve in Africa. My inability to buy clothing didn't affect the popular and thin's ability to fit into whatever items they wanted. My social inequity didn't affect their desire to flaunt themselves to a world that I wasn't privileged enough to be a part of. Truthfully, if they had any dignity or real friends at all, then someone should have told them to stop pouring themselves into those pants and halter tops about a size and a half ago. If they were going to create a visual fiasco, then I could not be held accountable for gawking at the scene that resulted. Lord knows they have had enough laughs at my expense.

I just could not understand how the world worked. After-school specials and hipster guidance counselors assured me that everyone was just lashing out over insecurities in themselves, and they only put me down to raise them up. But what were they all so insecure about? I wasn't seeking them out for verbal attacks. I hoped that it was caused by their insecurities, because if not, then what? Is it possible that they were just that cruel? Did they actually believe the value and worth of others around them was so low? Were their own lives not happy enough that they found it necessary to ruin and manipulate mine?

I was tired of failing at everything and reaching out for nothing. I prayed as I was told I should, but I never got an answer. Honestly, with all of the terrible things that were going on throughout the world, I was sure that one fat kid's inability to cure his addiction to fried dough was the last thing God needed to worry about. In the meantime... God if you are listening:
Please help me.

Chapter 10:

When You Can No Longer See Your Feet, You Have Gained So Much More Than Just the World

Have you ever laughed at someone so much you feel like you should thank them for the good times you've had at their expense? Even further, have you ever watched someone fail so miserably at something that it bypasses funny and just becomes sad? I felt I was becoming that person. It seemed that with each passing day, I had less and less control over myself and my actions. I was grateful that I reached for sandwiches rather than razor blades, but by that point, I question which lifestyle cut deeper. I ate because it was the only thing that calmed my emotions, but I was emotional because of my romance with food. I was overwhelmed with the guilt of it all. It wasn't just affecting my thought process; it dictated how I reacted in everyday situations. The last thing I wanted was my social life to end up like my closet, seemingly full, but lacking substance.

As a last-ditch effort to have any form of connection, I joined any social group that needed to meet a member quota. I applied my desire to create by designing and building backgrounds for our high school musicals. I used my mathletic ability to help the library club shelf returns. While sorting books by decimals was not the most amusing way to spend a study hall, they never talked down to me or made fun of me, so I guessed it was an upgrade. After a few months of building musical backdrops and hanging around those acting types, my own "acting" ability was inadvertently noticed. Some of the lesser-known drama club talents found my "Fat Like A Muse" mentality amusing and asked if I would help write the junior varsity Christmas play. Desperate for any form of connection, I jumped at the chance. (Figuratively of course, I can't imagine that I had any type of vertical in that condition. Well, except for NBA Jamz, but I digress). I, brimming with excitement, could not wait to add my perspective to a story that upheld a positive overweight stereotype.

Time however, would reveal different plans. As the story evolved, it became less about an incredible fat guy being the hero and more about love and romance.

I tried my best to offer the same funny fat kid comic relief that earned me the right to be there in the first place, but no one seemed to care once onstage romance was involved. The girls wanted a love story and the guys supported the girls in hopes that it would help them write a love story of their own. When writing nights turned into read-throughs and read-throughs turned into after-hour one-on-ones, my presence quickly became unnoticed. Once again, the musical chairs of love left me without a place to sit. Another social situation fell through thanks to the *Rochford* condition.

With waning options, I fazed myself back into the library's graces. Little did I know it would offer me the opportunity to audition for our school's puppetry club. I seriously considered it for a week or so, but once I saw the limited space behind the curtain, it became abundantly clear that I was too large for the smaller circumference of a puppet stage.

My life was turning into case study for the greatest amount of wasted potential. Believe it or not, up until that point, I had always believed that my eating was only a phase. I always thought someone or something would enter my life and replace my dependency for food with love and vigor. Since the time spent in the library gave me more of a relationship with Hemmingway than it did with Mary Ann, I began to doubt that love would ever find me.

Realizing that it never would, I turned further inward as my stomach turned further outward. Passing the point of surrender, standard self-medication was no longer satisfying. I no longer WANTED to have food, I NEEDED to have food.

I started sneaking off whenever I could to have eating contests with myself. I broke personal records at Mexico Bell by way of ten Santa Fe beef gorditas washed down with 64 ounces of Mt. Precipitation and finished off with a warm caramel empanada. When it came to snacking, I was an equal opportunity employer. My consumptional training forced me to think inside the bun.

The 20 Chicken Pacnugget challenge was no match for me. I consumed them all with room to spare for a large soda and two apple pies. The crowning glory had to be the Bettsies 99 cent value menu meal combo. I started off with a three-stack bacon cheeseburger with extra mayonnaise, girthy-sized with an order of chicken nuggets. Once the meal was consumed, I put the star on the tree by way of a 32-ounce Frothy. For me, it was a failsafe way to supplement emotional emptiness with caloric abundance. All I had to do was sacrifice my emotional dignity.

Months of apathetic binge eating transformed a kid with big dreams and aspirations into a 330 pound, 5 foot 8 shell of an individual. With summer quickly approaching, my parents started to plan what they believed might be our last family vacation. My sister was now in college, and they sensed that it was only a matter of time before they lost their baby girl to adulthood and wanted to seize one last opportunity for family time.

As my parents mapped the trip, they kept coming back to beach-centered destinations.

Mom, why do you keep choosing beach destinations?

> *Jeremy, you love beaches.*
> *Don't you remember*
> *Kyle and the great time you*
> *two had together?*

Mom, that was literally 8 years ago.

Why is it that parents only remember what they want to remember? Yes, granted, I USED to love the beach. But the larger I became, the greater my disdain for aquatic activities (i.e., swimming, beaches, attractive people wearing less than they should) became. In my younger days, before I knew what shame was, I loved the water. I loved to swim. I loved the beach. I absolutely loved it. Little did I know that it was actually buoyancy that I loved.

The fond memory my mother spoke of occurred when I was eight years old during one of my father's psychological conventions. While nestled in the Pocono Mountains, I befriended a like-minded eight-year-old kid named Kyle, who also LOVED water. Our hotel was adjacent to a lake, which was fully equipped by the resort with slides and diving boards. It was amazing. We tried our best to get as much air off of the diving boards as we could in the hopes that it would propel us to the bottom of the lake. We measured our success by whoever could grab the most seaweed while underwater. Well, I guess it would technically be lakeweed, however, lakeweed doesn't sound nearly as enchanting. Nevertheless.

My mother and I remembered that vacation so vividly because of how pure it was. We disconnect when she perceived my youthful state as present tense. She also failed to realize how self-conscious I had become. My awareness had heightened. I accepted that men were not designed to have cup sizes, so for the betterment of those around me, I kept my shirt on at all costs. Paramount to upholding this public service was staying away from any deliberate reason to take my shirt off. Reasons such as a family vacation that revolve around aquatic activities.

My mother, however, somehow looked past most of my faults and insecurities to only see the awesome (thanks, mom), never quite noticed this paradigm shift. Because of that (and parental rule), my weeks of resistance turned into hours staring out of the car window as I counted the mile markers that would lead us towards the Jersey shore.

Upon arrival, my sister wanted to head straight to the beach while I wanted nothing more than to hermitize myself in the hotel room to avoid any beach sociality. Against my will, I was parentally forced out to *enjoy* my boardwalk vacation. Nothing holds a place in my heart quite like the sweet aroma of the Jersey shore. As bad as the coast smells, the Garden State fragrance was merely a precursor to the perspiration dripping off of me thanks to the half mile marathon it took just to get to the boardwalk.

As we walked up the stairs to the main concourse, my sister took a deep breath as if to announce to the world that she had arrived. I, on the other hand, took a series of short breaths to announce that I would need medical attention if those cardiovascular episodes continued. If ever there was a visual manifestation of sibling disconnect, it was that very moment. My sister stood in the foreground as a beacon of self-confidence, radiating like the sunlight itself. As for me, I began to look around for the nearest arcade to hide in. I campaigned my sister with 15 minutes of wet blanketing until she decided to leave me to myself. The only condition was that we meet back together at that location as soon as the sun began to set.

Fawning over my victory, I claimed the nearest bench as though I had just invaded it. Finally, I got a chance to sit down. Scanning the area, my eyes noticed two things worthy of my attention. The first was a seaside candy shop and the second was a NASCAR-themed go-kart track. NASCAR? Yeah, I love it and I have no idea how it happened. One could theorize that wearing all of those racing shirts so tightly for so long eventually allowed the love of the sport to transfer from fabric to anatomy. But that's a lousy explanation because it doesn't even make sense. I guess the truth of it was that NASCAR seemed to have a large demographic, and considering I was not a fan of twicely named motorcycles; I aspired to find any acceptance or identity that I could. Call it shenanigans, but it was how I genuinely felt.

Deciding that the seductive call of sugar was far too loud to ignore, I promptly waddled over to the candy store. I passed through the door and felt instantaneously at home, except for how ironically small the aisles were. I assumed that pier-front real estate was expensive because of how small the store was. That, or possibly the owner underestimated the size of their demographic.

Forging ahead, I mentally perused which goodies I would consume. I threw down a five spot as I approached the counter and after a few minutes of pointing and clarifying, I was on my way. A few hundred paces in the distance was the sound of rolling thunder, well, technically it was the roaring lawnmower engines that powered the go-karts around the track.

I followed my ears to the observation deck that allowed the spectators to watch the cars circle around. As the cars were taking turns loading and unloading new racers, I noticed lines of my peers were waiting and enjoying their lives. They were smiling, flirting, and seemed truly happy. I was lost between the hum of the engines and the hopeless ideal that I could possibly find that form of happiness. I knew it was possible, but not in my condition. I raised the pound and a half of gelatinous joy and cursed its existence. In the same breath, I held it closer as it was the only support structure that hadn't let me down.

Halfway between a smile and a tear, I stood there observing the track and its festivities until twilight faded into darkness. Being true to my word, I made my way back to the bench to meet up with my sister. We walked to the condo we were staying in and upon entering the door, I kissed the air conditioned perfection and headed straight to bed.

I arose the next morning with the sun shining through the window, straight into my face. I begrudgingly sat up to notice my mother was the only other person awake. I stumbled over to the kitchen table to join her. After engaging in some groggily dialogue, we went out to the balcony and finished watching the sunrise. I told my mom about the candy store and go-karts. I affirmed the need to go back to both of them. In doing so, I asked what the family itinerary was. She told me that the day's schedule included a trip to the beach coupled with a lighthouse visit or two. Once we had all the pictures we could handle, we would return to shower up for dinner and then head over to the boardwalk.

It seems like a great plan,
what do you think?

If by boardwalk you mean go-karts, then yes,
 I think it is a fantastic plan.

Fine. You can do go-karts.

Yes!

Once everyone else awoke and got dressed, we put my mom's plan into action. While I need not remind you of my ongoing disdain for beaches, I want you to know my mother's itinerary created a brand new adversary: lighthouses. Really? Yes, really! I know what you are thinking. "Jeremy, how could these beacons of hope and direction to sea captains the world over ignite such righteous discontent?" Let me tell you. First of all, to be visible from hundreds of miles off of the coast, the houses need to tower multiple stories high.

While I fully accept that, I cannot accept the sleight of engineering that allowed these towering structures to withstand gale-force winds without proper elevator equipment. Forget the overweight and under athletic, how do you think our handicapped friends feel about this? That's busch-league, lighthouses. Absolutely busch-league. Coming to terms with the inevitable stair scaling is one thing. It's an entirely different set of emotions to overcome when it is realized just how small the stairwells are once inside. Adding insult to injury, the slopes are ridiculously steep. Knocking that to-do off of my mother's vacation list, it was time to grab a bite to eat and then walk over to the boardwalk. There was no way to conceal my excitement once I heard the roar of the go-karts. It was enough to put my own little motor into overdrive. That was the fastest I walked in years.

I beat them all to the entrance and promptly grabbed my place in line. My parents told my sister and I that they would be waiting for us at the spectator area. While waiting for what seemed like an eternity, I begin to look around at all of the different people in line with us. I wondered what these people were thinking about. I wondered if they were as happy as they seemed. I wondered why half of them looked like they didn't want be there. Do you think they were faking a lack of excitement?

Thinking about other people made me start to ask more questions. Things like, "Why is it that the closer attractive people get to water, the less clothing they feel they need to wear?" and "Why would you pretend to not be excited about go-karts?" Come on, really? Go-karts are awesome! Go-karts are like Sugar Ray and Fall Out Boy. No one wants to admit to liking what they do, but they keep selling albums, don't they? Numbers do not lie, my friends.

A couple of self-contemplations and sibling conversations later, we found ourselves standing at the front of the line. I scanned the remaining cars, and of course, the one I wanted was taken. I was okay with that; I had a second choice picked out from the recon I did the night before. I walked over at a fire drill's pace and wedged myself into the kart's roll cage. In doing so, I completely misgauged my dissent and received an unwelcome **hello** from the seatbelt lever. Upon digging that out, I adjusted my girth to get as comfortable as possible. After maneuvering around this cocoon of a cockpit in attempts to fasten my seatbelt, I was left with the realization that the two ends were not coming together. I mean, they weren't even close.

I wiggled around with such fervor that I unknowingly summoned the attendant to assist me. She reassuringly told me to relax and let her take care of it. She was sweet. She was also attractive, so I believed she was being personable because it was her job. She waited until I was comfortably settled and began to buckle me in....well...attempted to buckle me in. After a couple minutes of us playing Twister with my seatbelt, she had not gotten any further with securing me into the seat than I had.

Then, without warning, she walked away. Not too far, just far enough away to think she was out of earshot. I could hear her angrily mumble something under her breath but could not quite make it out. She placed her head in her hand and stood there for what seemed like eternity. Why was she not buckling me in? Why was this taking so long? Why was everybody staring at me? Then she came back, and before I could say a word, she looked me dead in the eye and said...

You know, if you just stop squirming
maybe we can wiggle it in.

I understand that.
I'm squirming because every time you push
down you're pinching a stomach roll.

Sir, this is no time for joking.
If we can't get this to lock, we can't let you ride.
I have been trying for the past 15 minutes,
so now is not the time to be funny.

I'm not trying to be funny,
you are physically hurting me!
Every time you push down you pinch
my skin and the harder you push,
the harder it is to breathe.

I'm sorry sir; there just is no other way.
Every time I get close, my fingers slip
from your sweat. Can you sweat less?

Are you serious? I'm uncomfortable as it is
and now people are gathering around because
of the scene were making.

I just don't know what I can do.
Hold on, let me get my boss.
"HEY RICHIE, CAN YOU COME HERE?"

129

Fantastic!?!

Yeah? What's the problem?

Well, this gentleman would like to ride the go-karts, however, we can't seem to get him to fit.

We'll that's not a problem.
We can seat him in the #22 car.
That car is reserved for our "huskier" guests.

Um...

What is it?

This is the #22 car.

Are you sure?

Yup.

Oh. Hmm… Well…

Is there some sort of extender we can use?

Um. Not really. No. Well, yes. But. Um.
For safety reasons they're already built into the #22 car.
Because of our insurance, we equipped at least
one car with a harness system built for
a...well...um...more "manly" man.

Sir? Are you okay?
You look like you're crying.

Oh me? Ha ha...no...it's just the sun.
Sunscreen, you know...the sweat...
in my eyes...heat...yeah. The sun.
 I'm fine.

Are you sure?

Yeah, (tear) fine.

Here. What if we
just pull this like this...

OH SNAPPP! COME ON!
OH MAN THAT HURTS!!!

Well if you would
just stop squirming…

I'M SQUIRMING BECAUSE
YOU ARE HURTING ME!!!

Sir, stop yelling!
You are the one who got us into this.
Well, actually you are the one who is
preventing us from getting you into this.

What?

Nothing.
It's just in all of my years of running this ride,
I have never seen this happen. Ever.
I just don't know what else to do.

So, what are you saying?

What I am saying is that in every summer I have
come to this boardwalk as a patron,
as a ride operator, and now as a manager ,
I have never seen anyone turned away from this ride
because they could not fit. Now I have to do just that.
Sir we have tried everything, and you are
not fitting into the safety harness. I'm sorry sir,
you are going to have to leave. Now, would you
please step this way as to not further hold up the line.

What!?! Are you serious!?!

Sir, I am really sorry.
But I have a line and you do not fit safely in the car.
I am very sorry, but I am going to have to ask you to leave.

In that very moment, everything I was or had ever
hoped to be, lay in motionless disbelief. My youth, my
innocence, and my desire to live had been reduced to nothing
more than a chalk outline buried within.

I walked out through the gates, past the crowd of my
peers, onlookers, and curious workers. In doing so, I was
greeted with a less than favorable exit. Words which cut deeper
than razorblades filled the air and landed upon me. Statements
of repulsion, which cannot be repeated without a parental
advisory, were spoken to me like it was commonplace. What
made this worse was that my parents were watching this unfold
from the bird's eye view up on the observation area.

What should have been a great memory for our entire family was now reduced to the most embarrassing day of my life. My parents met me at the exit with every intention of consolation. I looked right through them and said I just wanted to go to the condo. With a brief hesitation, they handed me the room key. I told them I would be there for the rest of our vacation. My mother attempted to follow me, but my father quickly pulled her back. He said, "Cath, you just need to let him go."

Walking past the aroma of the candy store sparked my ever-wandering attention. However, this time was different. Instead of wanting to wrap myself in the comfort it would provide, I wanted to scream at the top of my lungs, "This is what you did to me!" As I looked upon my reflection in the window, I could not muster a sound. With all the rage of a broken spirit, bloodshot eyes, and tear-stained shirt, I knew the reason for all of this was me. I was the one who did this, no one else.

I carried myself up the stairs of our vacation home, opened the door, and buried my face in a pillow. Then I cried. I cried as loud as my lungs would allow. When I was all out of tears, I started screaming. I screamed at the mirror for reflecting what I had become. I screamed at my parents' bed (as through they were there) for allowing me to turn into this. Finally, I turned my attention to God. I screamed at him the loudest and the longest. I screamed until my voice was gone.

"Why God? Why? Why, if you *love* people so much, would you allow things like this to happen? Why can't you just fix me? Why can't you fix *your* creation?" I was so angry. Once I lost my voice, I was fortunate enough to regain my tears. Once they both left me, I started to look around the room for any and all ways to end my misery. While there were many viable options, sharp objects, elevated heights, and unstable riptides all at my disposal, I just couldn't do it. Ironic, for all of the self-destruction I had enjoyed over the past 16 years, I just could not kill myself. The one thing I should be good at, I was not. It seemed that the story of my life was one incomplete after another.

So, as I had done so many times before, I lay face down on the floor in tearful contemplation. I rationalized that suicide was not the best option. I knew it would solve my problem quickly, but it would have created so many more for so many other people. Truthfully, that just wouldn't have been fair. I thought of my parents. Why should they have to suffer through the pain of burying their child? As a parent, that's the worst thing one could suffer. I thought about the scar it would have been on my sister's social reputation. She would forever be the girl with the broken family. That's not fair to her.

My affirmation that suicide was not the best option did very little to establish what would be. This was the only life I had lived, and an overweight lifestyle was all I had known. I was far beyond a diet cola fix.

As I lay there playing solutional hopscotch in my head, I noticed my family making their way up the stairs. They did their best to pretend nothing had happened. I had no problem acting dumb and playing along. The rest of my vacation, I put on the fake smile that I had become so accustomed to wearing. Inside, I wanted nothing more than to be anywhere but there.

Chapter 11:

Caloric Bankruptcy

I always questioned New Jersey t-shirts that claim "Only the Strong Survive," but after that weekend, I clearly understood the slogan. There will always be a place in my heart for the Garden State; I just hoped that I would never have to see it again.

The past seven days had been the longest and most painful of my life. However, what was a living hell for me might actually have been an answered prayer for others. In the proper context, I can see how weight loss is similar to religion. The further you push it upon someone who is not ready or willing to receive it, the further you push them away. However, when the heart of the afflicted is broken enough to actively seek redemption, true transformation will be sought out. Our vacation not only left me broken, but it also removed the proverbial veil from my eyes. I could no longer ignore the consequences of my actions.

Clearly, there were a lot of changes that needed to be made in my life. Fortunately, the 8-hour ride home provided plenty of time to consider every available option. I always romanticized a gastric bypass approach for weight loss. The idea of losing mass quantities of weight while doing little to no exercise warmed my heart. But in my case, I couldn't justify the risk. I had the rest of my life ahead of me, and the possibility of losing it on an operating table because I would rather take a scalpel to the abdomen than a lap around the track seemed fairly immature.

Realistically, it would have taken less effort to commit to a gym for a year than it would have to deal with the entire post op, physical therapy, and re-conditioning I would have endured while rehabbing my surgically pieced together midsection. So I could suffer without stitches or a co-pay, or I could suffer with a myriad of scars, complications, and traumas. I don't know about you, but my mother always said that being stabbed is a bad idea, even if it's from the hands of a professional.

Joking aside, my stomach wasn't really the problem. My stomach was merely a visual sign that I wouldn't stop eating. I didn't understand what "full" was, and somehow along the way, an overstuffed stomach had become associated with romance. No amount of surgery was going to fix that. Truthfully, if I did have the bypass without taking care of my mental dependencies, then it would have only been a matter of time until I pushed my stomach back out again.

No, bypass was a bad option because it would waste both time and money. I moved on and began sizing up my corporate weight loss options such as Metabolic Fast or West Coast Weight Loss. After reviewing what they had to offer, I believed that none of them would work for me.

My hesitation was this: why are B-rate celebrities and former athletes selling me their product instead of success stories? Wouldn't you think if those spokespeople had better career opportunities they would have taken them? Since it appeared that they did not, I could only imagine the amounts of free time they had to devote solely to exercise.

I mean, how much weight could I lose if it was my job?

It just seemed like these programs cared more about selling products than they did providing weight loss solutions; which explained why their office job postings always required a degree in sales and business rather than health and wellness. How did I know this? There was free internet in the library, and Career Constructer was one of the only sites that wasn't parentally controlled. Plus, if I told Mrs. Thomas that I was doing career research for when I graduated, she didn't make me dust the shelves when there were no books to return.

Back to corporate weight loss. My mother had been on and off of "Weight Observers" so many times that I lost track. The only thing I actually learned from their program was how to manipulate their points system as much as I manipulated my parents. I always had to question why a program designed for permanent results and progressive independence also encouraged a lifetime membership. It seemed as though they were trying to grant me a degree that would expire the moment I stepped off of campus. So, I ruled them out.

What about the Lap-Band®,
that idea seems solid?

No, it's a non-permanent form of the bypass,
which once again, doesn't solve my problem.

Hmm. You are running
out of logical options.

I know, and we still have three hours left to drive.

Well how about illogical options?

Like what? Those pills again? That's stupid.
You saw how that ended up. I became cranky,
 I developed insomnia. Then when it didn't work,
 I lashed out at others. No, I think if I am going to buy
into some form of corporate lie, I will buy into the
"You can do whatever you set your mind to" lie.

How is that a lie?

Because it is. I have tried for years to lose weight
 and all it did was yo-yo back and forth, leaving me
 even fatter than when I started. It is a statement
that promises hope and delivers failure.

Tried for years to lose weight?
*NO, that is the exact **opposite** of what you have done.*
You could write a book about all the times you ran
away from weight loss and did something
ridiculously drastic just so you could avoid it.
And as far as failure, Jeremy, failure implies that
you have tried something. Jeremy, you have
NEVER tried to lose weight. EVER!

But what about?

EVER!

Are you always trying to be a downer?

No, Jeremy, you always do this.
You get so caught up in the latest and
the greatest to the point that you
waste all of your time preparing to start,
but you never actually start anything.
That is why a statement like,
"You can do whatever you set your mind to"
bothers you. It's because all you see are
empty promises without results.
What I see is you getting so excited
about what could happen,
that you never commit the time to make it happen.
It's this perpetual cycle of you about to start,
but you never do. So you really haven't failed at anything,
it's just that you have never really tried
hard enough to actually begin something.

Is that really what's going on here?

Yeah, you don't see it because you are living it.
But I, as a part of your subconscious,
get to see it all, as well as the motives.
Think of me as a critic.
I don't actually contribute anything of substance,
I merely make fun of the failure of those who do.
The beauty, is if you take that failure, or lack of even trying,
and you use it as passion to prove others wrong,
then you will accomplish things greater than you can imagine.

I guess that logic rules out all of these fake diet pills and fads.

Knowing me, books probably won't work. I mean, who really gets anything substantial out of a weight loss book anyway? Most of them are shelved in personal growth sections, which is ironic because it is not our inability to grow that has us seeking a book on weight loss in the first place. So what is the solution then, overly-critical subconscious?

Logic, Jeremy, logic.
Take all of the things that have
put you in this state and seek out the exact opposite.
You don't know the first thing about eating right.
Find somebody who does.
You sneak food in ridiculous amounts;
surround yourself with accountability.
You don't exercise because you don't know how.
Find someone who does. Learn from them.
Jeremy, weight loss is not rocket science.
But making it mean something to you is.

So, basically if I stop chasing safety
and actually apply myself for once,
I can achieve great things?

Yep.

While in that moment it sounded a lot like "You can do whatever you set your mind to," hearing it from a different voice gave that perspective a validity I felt it had been lacking. Maybe my mind was playing tricks on me during that car ride, but I felt as though weight loss might be attainable.

By the time I was ready to lay my head down and catch a quick car nap, we were almost in our driveway. While unpacking the luggage, I asked my parents if we could have a townhall meeting the next day to discuss the life changes that I felt needed to occur. They cordially agreed, and for once in my life, I went to bed with a defined sense of purpose and a desire to embrace tomorrow.

Once the sunrise gave way to mid-morning sunlight, I rolled out of bed for the lunchtime meeting with my parents. Sitting down over a nice bologna sandwich and a side of conviction, we discussed the lower points of the vacation and what we felt could be learned from them. It took nearly half an hour of deliberation to conclude that any weight loss of mine would need professional intervention. Sharing my feelings and satire with them on corporate weight loss, they assured me that we would seek out a physician-supervised, medically sound program.

Options were plenty, but my parents decided to schedule an appointment with the Bariatric Weight Loss Center. As the week drew to a close, I found myself in their Squirrel Hill office to meet with the staff. We went over the normal formalities; why I was there, what I hoped to learn from this experience, how many days a week I planned to weigh in. Once the informational meetings were wrapped up, we began to discuss my weight loss meal plan.

As a part of my overall health, my water consumption needed to increase from almost nothing to 84 ounces a day. A B vitamin complex was administered to jumpstart my metabolism. The biggest component of my program would focus on exercise to not only speed up the weight loss metabolization process, but also to burn away the fat I had packed on for so long.

By the end of the first week, I had lost nine pounds. After the second week, I was down another 10. By the first day of school, I was almost under 300 pounds. I couldn't believe the success I was having.

Everything worked flawlessly until the politics of the school lunchroom reminded me that life still had no place for the overweight, not even those seeking reform. While waiting in line, I noticed the familiar smell of scented body sprays mixed with greasy mystery meat. Was it a burger, was it meatloaf, was it avoidable? I was not sure, but I was about to find out.

Approaching the serving station, I asked the lunch lady if there was a healthier option than what was being served. Her eyes glared at me through her drooping hairnet as she sternly said, "You know, if you don't like what we are serving for lunch today you can always go to yesterday's line and see if they have any sloppy joes left. If that doesn't do it for you, you are more than welcome to bring your lunch from home."

But you see, that was part of the problem. Food designed to sit in a non-refrigerated environment for five hours was what helped get me in such poor nutritional health to begin with. On top of that, there was no room for any of those preservative-filled pre-packaged foods on my meal plan.

So there I was, seeking something better for my health and my best option was a poorly cooked replication of a cheeseburger. I mean, the cheese wasn't even melted. It was just lying there between the bun and the meat like an un-firm handshake, useless, limp, and almost pouting. I walked away from the line and over to my lunch table. I put my head in my arms and began to contemplate. It was no wonder I was as fat as I was. My options were terrible. I never expected four ounces of baked chicken with six ounces of steamed asparagus, but when a fat kid has to argue with the lunch lady to get a salad, there is a flaw in the system.

Maintaining my meal plan seemed like an exercise in futility. Those first two months were great because I had control over my food options as well as my schedule. Now, I was at the mercy of The Czar of Lunch Lady Land.

I did anything and everything possible to get my mind off of that day's failure. As I took my lunch lady's advice a little more personally than I should have, I began to think how I could make my allotted food work within the confines of a packed lunch.

I tried my best to eat the five-hour locker inhabited vegetables, but I just didn't have the patience (or the stomach) for lukewarm, soggy carrots. I began to skip meals, and even worse, binge on school lunches. All of my inconsistencies began a cycle where I would gain one pound, lose two, gain four pounds, and lose six.

After having initial success, there seemed to be no way to sustain any weight loss program. I just didn't have the freedom I needed to be loyal to it. Maybe in another life or when I have the freedom of schedule, but at that moment, I just couldn't do to it.

And so you are quitting again.
I knew you would. Pansy.

What?

You heard me.

How can you even say that?
You of all people have a first-hand view
 of the fact that I have no control over this.

> *Yes, you cannot control the fact that*
> *one of a thousand doctor-recommended*
> *weight loss programs doesn't*
> *fit into your circumstances,*
> *but you do have control over the fact*
> *that you are choosing to quit*
> *rather than use the brain that God*
> *gave you for something other than*
> *destroying your life.*

So what exactly are you suggesting?

> *Jeremy, I have said it before and I*
> *will say it again: weight loss is not rocket science.*
> *Weight loss at its core is a numbers game.*
> *It is no different than getting out of debt.*
> *You need to eat less, and you need to do more.*
> *The problem is that the human condition that*
> *got us here has made the space between*
> *being ready to accept that truth and being*
> *ready to act upon it so insurmountable,*
> *that it never is surmounted.*

*You, on the other hand, are the exact opposite.
You are ready to lose weight and want
a structured program, but the one in a
thousand that you have to follow
doesn't work in your schedule right now.
Jeremy, the honest truth is that
you will always face obstacles
but as a counter point, you will always have a
weight loss solution that will work for you.
You just have to realize it.
What you need to do is take the program
the doctor has given you and stop asking
"What can I eat?" and start to ask
"Why are they making me eat this?"*

And with another bit of shared wisdom, sarcasm, and momentary flashback, my subconscious was right. It was time to stop asking the "whats" and start asking the "whys." One of the most convenient things about being a high school senior was the amount of unnecessary downtime I had. I never realized just how much of my day was wasted by staring aimlessly at a wall.

I figured instead of looking busy and wasting time, I would actually get busy and seize it. I began to analytically pick apart my weight loss program. I researched the foods that were on my OK list and compared them to the foods I used to eat. I started a list of all of the behaviors I practiced prior to my program and all of the changes that were mandated. I counted calories, grams, and ounces. Which by the way, how did OZ become the abbreviation for ounce? There isn't even a Z in the word. It doesn't make sense and it doesn't matter. What mattered was that I came up with the solution for my obesity problem.

How so? I applied common sense to all areas of my life. I started to monitor exactly what I was consuming. The first thing I did was start a journal. In that journal, I created a nutritional budget. For me, it was an act of accountability. If I was going to eat it, I was going to have to write it. If I had to write it, I would have to explain it. Those pages acted as a resolution of freedom or a diary of shame. Either way, it was honest.

I started to look at weight loss as a path of least resistance. Could I eat whatever I wanted to? Sure, but I also had to admit to myself that I could not expect to lose weight with a weight maintenance mentality. Was a bottle of Mountain Precipitation permissible? Yes, but it was 400 calories. In the grand scheme of things, that was a full meal if I planned correctly. I consistently found myself asking the question, what is the path of least resistance? Is bottle of Mountain Precipitation worth having instead of a sandwich? Is an ice cream cone really worth an entire meal? It became a war of common sense rather than unattainable results. Finally, I was in control.

Now I know what you are thinking. Jeremy, I am glad that calorie counting worked for you, but I just don't have the time/patience/desire to do that. Okay, that's fair; I completely understand where you are coming from. However, let me ask you this: do you count your money? Do you monitor how much money you have in your account versus how much debit you owe? Why?

For me the answer was simple: the amount of money one has controls the type of life one can live. Right? Is it not living that allows one to be able to make money? Likewise, if your health to debt ratio runs out...so would your money, right? If you are dead or incapacitated due to weight, it hardly matters all the money you counted. It only makes sense to take care of what makes the money, before you worry about counting your money.

It was about taking responsibility for my actions and knowing what I was consuming, instead of blindly stuffing myself. I took this mentality and I fully embraced it. Everything became a choice. I finally had a declaration of independence over food. I was no longer the victim; I was the one in control. If I only had thought like this earlier, how much of my life would I have not wasted? Why are the simplest riddles the hardest to solve?

Chapter 12:

Start Living or Die Trying

Among the many things I brought back from our Jersey vacation, other than tear-stained eyes and a feeling of self-loathing, there was one redeeming souvenir that needs to be mentioned. **B**efore the **G**o-**K**art **I**ncident, now officially recognized **BGKI**, I purchased a limited edition, officially licensed Eric Cartman South Park t-shirt. Now, most cartoon t-shirts (and NASCAR t-shirts for that matter) tend to get way too busy and obnoxious with their designs. Not this one. No, the simplicity of this shirt was just too normal to pass up. It had one small logo on the front, one large logo on the back. Most importantly, there was no annoying catchphrase that would be culturally irrelevant four months after I purchased the shirt, printed anywhere on it.

However, the problem was this: while I was a huge Eric Cartman fan in **BGKI** times, it was now in the **AGKI** or **A**fter the **G**o-**K**art **I**ncident era, and I could no longer endorse the fat kid qualities that Eric Cartman embodied. He is loud-mouthed, obnoxious, insulting, and while you were not able to miss him, most would go out of their way to avoid a person like that.

In the before times (**BGKI**), I would have done anything for attention, so having adoration for Cartman made sense to me. Problem was, I no longer wanted to be known as the fat kid who was angry at the world. I was already avoided for no other reason than being an orb-like obstacle to those walking in the hallway. Truthfully, I didn't want to be remembered for any of that. In my condition, rigorous weight loss could literally have killed me. I would rather be remembered for trying something than forgotten for doing nothing. If I was ever going to be the change I wanted to see in this world, then I needed to become the change I wanted to see in myself.

Once I got home, I found that Cartman shirt, symbolizing whom I no longer wanted to be. I cut the sleeves off and committed to wear it as my weight loss uniform. I wanted it to serve as a reminder that until my weight was gone, I would forever carry the burden of misrepresentation, judgment, and hate from an outside world that didn't care to understand the heartbreak of being overweight. The laughing world may never have the desire to change their opinion of the overweight. That's fine. I'll change it for them.

Now, while I admit that was a captivating story in all forms of literary expression, it serves absolutely no propose in addressing the fact that I still needed to find a way to work my weight off. Looking back, I often wonder how my journey would have played out if it started in present day. I say that because there seems to be a gym on every corner now. But I digress. Because this was a few years back in the day (which contrary to popular belief, was not a Wednesday), my options were limited to the high school facilities, Carnegie Library of Homestead gymnasium, or buying my own home workout equipment.

Each one had their drawback. The drawbacks to working out at the high school facility were self-evident. If I decided to work out at home, I would have to deal with the awkwardness of parental encouragement, which is sometimes more annoying than it is helpful. My father, bless his heart, had every best intention when he purchased discount exercise equipment. For some reason, he never got the point that it was inexpensive for a reason. At one time or another, our basement was filled with manually powered treadmills, some Nordic-looking apparatus, and cable-based weight restraints. These were all manually powered and were so painstaking to assemble, that once you did, the last thing you wanted to do was look at them again. They were not my friends. So our inexpensive workout equipment matured into really expensive clothing hangers.

I needed something that was going to work with me, not against me. This was my time to follow through, which left my only viable option as the Carnegie Library gym. Being one with a nerdy disposition, I already knew where the library was. I had spent numerous hours there, but it never occurred to me until I saw the advertisement that a gymnasium was right upstairs. I had to see for myself just how useful those facilities might be. I saddled up the minivan and drove on down. I only wanted a tour, but after the nice elderly gentleman told me they offered a student discount, I signed up on the spot. I guess that's my lineage coming out. I saw a potentially useless item or service at a discount price and I couldn't resist.

So it was. Signed and sealed. Jeremy Rochford, the next day of the rest of your life was about to begin. School came, went, and for once in my life, food wasn't at the forefront of my thought process. All day my mind was focused on going to the gym. I could not wait to show people how wrong they were for giving up on me. I was so afraid and yet so excited at the exact same time.

I walked up the stairs, shoulders straight, head held high as I passed through the doors. Making my way up one final flight, I found myself face to face with the receptionist, who was male. Maybe receptor would be a more masculine term for him. It doesn't matter. I showed him my card and proceeded. As I passed through the poorly lit corridor that connected the outside world to this valley that overlooked the shadow of death, I promise you, I feared no evil. I made sure my Walkman was cocked and loaded, ready to disengage any negative emotions with the flick of a finger. I pressed play to allow "Bulls on Parade" the right to usher in a new legacy of what could only be known as:

JEREMY ROCHFORD, VERSION 2.0. UPGRADE. BETA

The fluorescent light nearly blinded me as the scenery went from cave-like to operating room in a matter of seconds. As I was greeted by an empty canvas in the form of a workout facility, I quickly realized that I had absolutely no idea what I was supposed to do next. I looked around the room; clearly there was a machine for every part of the body that would need to be worked. Being as large as I was, I knew any of them would have been beneficial. But they all looked so potentially painful and awkwardly confusing. Fortunately, I was the only one there, so no one noticed me staring without aim. I knew, however, that it would not last for long. I had to make a plan.

I was about to go over to the chest weights when out of the corner of my eye an angelic piece of grey and black machinery caught my attention. It called to me with an intimate voice that until now, only frosting had known. It was indeed a treadmill. Right next to it was a stationary bike. While not knowing the first thing about weight training, I did know how to walk. Even further, I knew how to ride a bike. I was now equipped to sculpt this body of mine.

*You make it sound so **epic**!*

Not now.

In haste, I propelled myself over to the treadmill. I stepped on it and began to enter my weight. Slowly, I watched the number climb from 155 to 300. Then it beeped. So I kept pressing. And it kept beeping, showing 300 all the while. Then it started to flash. Then I started to swear. "What? What is this? What do you mean it won't go past 300 pounds? So what happens now? Have I reached the level where I am too fat to be fat? Am I too overweight to work out? Did I break it just by stepping on it? You've got to be kidding me." I thought to myself.

I fired back. "You know what? You are probably one of those treadmills who waits around for a nice high school girl with a slender tan behind wearing cute little boy shorts to work out on you. Well guess what Lyfe Fitness? You're getting a fat and sweaty one today! Deal with it!"

Once I came to terms with the fact that I just argued with an inanimate treadmill over its gender preference, I decided to enter 300 pounds and move on.

Maybe it was the anger of the aforementioned argument, but I ambitiously set the timer to 30 minutes. I was on my way. Five minutes went by and I decided to BAM, take it up a notch. At the ten-minute mark, I was dying for air. You never truly realize how out of shape you are until something else determines how hard you have to work. By the 15-minute mark I had to BAM ...retract it down a notch. Once 20 minutes rolled around, it looked as though a rain cloud had hovered above and released sheets of sweat over me. After 25 minutes, I was holding onto the side rails for dear life, and when it finally hit 30 minutes and decelerated for cool-down, I honestly could not feel my legs underneath me.

Once cool-down was complete and I regained feeling in my lower extremities, I walked over to the water fountain to get a drink. On my way over, my reflection stopped me dead in my tracks. This was the first time in 30 minutes that I had actually looked in the mirror.

Words cannot do justice to the visual fiasco I beheld. As it turned out, a very large high school student sweating himself into shape while wearing a white t-shirt bears a strikingly similar resemblance to a very well-endowed female college student participating in a wet-t shirt contest. And while there has been no scientific evidence as to why men have nipples, I was convinced it was to embarrass me to death at that very moment.

By the time my eyes were able to disengage from the mirror, I noticed that I was not the only one pondering my nipple query. To this day, I have never seen such confused looks. Unbeknownst to me, three other people were also staring at me in wonderful amazement. Their eyes affixed on me as though they just witnessed a 20-car pileup in which every car was destroyed by flames, yet every single person walked away from the wreckage all the while finding deserving homes for 20 baby puppies. It just didn't make sense to anyone. The scene was beyond comprehension.

Yet, there I stood at the center of everyone's attention. I looked back at my reflection and all I could think was, "If they're not laughing at me for this, then they would be laughing at me for something else." Memories flashed back from when desks collapsed under my weight in both eighth and ninth grades. The day that my family and I had to move from the booth at our favorite Steak & Sea house to a table and chairs because I could no longer wedge myself into family-style seating. Lest we forget the go-karts.

No. No more. It ends here. I had been made fun of for killing myself for the past 16 years. I would not be made fun of for turning my life around. I was through with crumbling inside every time something embarrassing like this happened. All I was trying to do was right a body that I had wronged for so many years. No mature person could shake his or her head at that. Not one.

As time began to move forward, I handled the rest of the situation so epically that to this day I have no idea how it occurred. As I wiped the sweat from my brow, I looked up at those who were around me. Looking back at the mirror and then looking back at them, I pointed in the direction of the cardio equipment and said, "Well.... the treadmill works." Smiling as I turned away, I felt a rush of freedom that I cannot explain. Walking out of the room I felt something that I had never felt before from the eyes of my peers. Respect.

I threw my gym bag into the back of the minivan, paused, and stood there for a moment. I had to make sure that what had just occurred actually happened. I looked up at the stars and tried to hold back my emotions. Try as I might, a few tears still fell from my eyes. Nothing amazing. No sobbing. Just joy. Just the feeling as though, for once in my life, everything would turn out okay.

I got in the car and had a hard time pulling away. I honestly did not want this feeling to end. I had lived a life of defeat for so long that I had forgotten what victory really felt like.

As I lay my head down to sleep that evening, I felt surrounded by the most euphoric peace that I had ever felt. I stared at the ceiling knowing that I had taken the first step of a journey that would define the rest of my life. When I said my goodnight prayers that evening, I remember thinking for first time, "I am truly thankful for the life that God has given me."

Chapter 13:

It's You and Me Cupcake: These Pants Aren't Big Enough For the Two of Us

(FLASHING) 6:00a.m.....BUZZ......BUZZ...BUZZ.....BUZZ.....

With the grace and poise of a gazelle, a shadowy mass sprawls towards an obnoxious buzzing alarmed apparatus with outstretched arms.

S-M-A-C-K!!!!! He makes contact with the alarm.

B-A-N-G!!!!! He also makes contact with the floor.

P-O-W!!!!!

S-H-A-Z-A-M!!!!!

UUUUUGGGGGHHHHHH! This floor is a lot harder than I remember it being. All right, I guess I better get up before this alarm clock decides to ring again.

Upsy - daisy.

Wait a minute.

Um....huh?

Why am I not moving?

I'm not paralyzed, am I?

No....that can't be possible.

I'm too young to be paralyzed.

Wait, that doesn't make sense. Age has nothing to do with the possibility that I may have jumped out of bed at such an angle that I may have broken something vital?

Hold on.

I can see my left hand. Can I see my right hand? (Head turns.) Okay. I can see that one, too. (Head turns back to face the ceiling.) I wonder if I can see my feet. Wait, never mind, I couldn't see my feet yesterday. All right, if I can move my neck then clearly I am not dead, but I wonder if I can feel or move my feet? (Feet wiggling successfully.) Sweet. Okay, if I can move and feel my feet, then paralysis is not the problem. So then what is?

What our hero had quickly forgotten is the cost of last night's moral victory with the treadmill came with the price of over-exhausting every muscle in his body. Since he worked them in ways they had never been worked before, Jeremy is experiencing a soreness he has never felt since. Silly boy.

What a minute here, was that all about?

You overdid it yesterday.

What?

You heard me.
You overdid it and now you are lying on the floor,
sore and discouraged.

Well, I'm definitely sore,
I'm hardly discouraged.

Not yet.
But you still have an entire
day of living to go through.
Give it time.

My loathing of you knows no end.

I peeled myself off of the floor and tried to wake up. I needed to shake off the haze of what just occurred as well as the flashback that explained it all. It took climbing down one household flight of stairs for my subconscious to declare itself victorious. On my way down to the shower, my parents asked me why I was limping so much. I assured them there was nothing to worry about, my limp was merely a byproduct of an effective workout program.

With that out of the way, I carried onward to the

shower. Turning the water on initiated another morning round of hokey pokey with the ever-alternating water temperatures. Apparently, the water heater had no sympathy for my soreness. After finding a rare moment of temperate stability, I let out a sigh of accomplishment while the warm water loosened my tense muscles.

That was the first time I could remember waking with sore abdominals due to muscular shrinkage. There had been plenty of times I woke up with side-splitting abs because I ate so much the night before that my stomach had to expand to accommodate it all. But not this time, this was a different kind of sore. This was the kind of sore that made you want to take on the world just to prove to them you could do it all over again.

My "wake up the voiceless" mentality quickly turned silent as self-proclamation turned into self-realization once first period required me to squeeze into a desk that was still way too small to accommodate my size. As you can imagine, squeezing out of it was just as unpleasant. Making my way down the hall towards the library, I passed a group of people who normally found their jollies in announcing my inadequacies. I lowered my head and waited for the fall. By the time I raised my head, I was already ten feet past and they had said nothing. Was it really true that confidence had the power to silence all critics?

I walked into the library and sat down to waste yet another study hall. Pulling out my weight loss pad, I began to journal last night's activities. I wrote down the awesome feeling of overcoming something that had been out of reach for so long. As I clicked out some more #2 lead, my mind wandered about the ramifications of my situation past, present, and future.

As my mind wondered about nothing at all, it also began contemplating something I never expected to think about, a topical classroom discussion. My psychology teacher suggested that geniuses act out in ways that are self-destructive because their above-average intelligence fails them in social situations.

This statement was offered to the class as a way to reflect on how we handle ourselves in our own social situations. If you have never heard of this theory, simply refer to the Tom Hanks movie "That Thing You Do." I feel there is very little legitimacy in that theory. While I do not consider myself a genius in any terms, I do believe if one is intelligent enough to be aware of their own aptitude, then inherently, they should be clever enough to apply their intellect in ways which are beneficial to their life, rather than destructive.

Furthermore, if said person is in fact a genius who willingly partakes in self-destructive behaviors, their genius should allow them to do so in a manner which allows them to avoid entrapment. Not just that, but also places them above suspicion. That is, of course, if said person is even a genius to begin with.

But I never believed my intelligence had any thing to do with my struggle. My struggles had always been with my emotional attachment to food and the desire to convince myself otherwise. It had never been an "Am I smart enough to overcome this?" issue; it had been an "Am I honest enough with myself to overcome this?" issue. One of the greatest deceptions I believed was that being overweight was my dirty little secret. How can something that draws so much public ridicule be considered a secret? I don't know, but it never stopped me from feeling like I just pulled off an amazing bank heist when I would sneak away to eat.

Interestingly, it was the feeling of the whole world watching me grow larger and larger that forced me to act out in the ways that made me overweight to begin with. I flipped the page of my journal and wrote down a list of all of the reasons I found it necessary to eat. In times where I felt sad, happy, depressed, overjoyed, celebratory, confused, ecstatic, bored, stressed, deprived, exhausted, lazy, awkward, disciplinary, nervous, habitual, afraid, relaxed, frustrated, self-conscious, angry, defiant, hopeless, broken, ineffective, lethargic, unknowing, fearful, needing to fill a void, unloved, hurt, needing to cope, wanting to be social, unable to resist the temptation of...

By the time the bell rang, I compiled nearly two pages of reasons I believed it was necessary to eat. Looking over the list, I realized that hunger was one of the last reasons listed. I mean, I literally listed 50 reasons I had to eat before hunger even showed up. How it is possible that the one true indicator of "it's time to eat" mattered so little to me?

As I made my way to the lunch table, eating was the last thing I could think about. I pulled out my food and just kind of stared at it. After listing the reasons I ate and realizing that hunger wasn't as important to me as 50 other things, my heart sank. I really felt as though food had betrayed me. It's like it made the promise of a better life by the way it made me feel and the way I perceived it, and when it came time for food and I to be happy together, it left me standing there with high blood pressure, susceptibility to type 2 diabetes, a weakened heart, and a broken sociality. I gave all of my love to food, and no matter how hard I tried to make it, food never loved me back.

For the first time in my life, I was no longer jealous of those who were able to eat what they wanted.

Bringing myself back to reality, it was hard for me to even eat the food in front of me. Hard as it was, I forced myself. I had also learned that starving oneself is only a recipe for failure. The human body does need fuel. It was my 4000 calories worth of food that I stuffed into 2000-calorie days that got me in trouble, not an apple.

For the rest of the day, my resentment towards food only became stronger. On the drive home past the former Munhall Hat-Trick, I wanted to yell at all three stops, "Look what you've done to me!" But I knew that it wasn't their fault, they were just being diligent business people. Convincing myself that eating four doughnuts a day was an acceptable form of anything should bear the brunt of any blame.

Once I committed to success, I found that success committed to me. Days turned into weeks and while there were peaks and valleys, my focus never shifted. One of the greatest surprises of my weight loss journey was my allegiance with the scale. I weighed myself twice a week, and I would count it once. Oh man. I never thought the day would come where I would like a scale. I used to hate the scale. I *HATED* it. However, after I ran out of journaling non-sensical reasons to eat, I began to dissect the reasons that I had declared war on scales the world over.

As I wrote what I thought would be a condemning declaration of just cause, I started to realize my hatred for the scale was merely a cover-up for personal non-achievement. Truthfully, the scale is an inanimate object. It can only reflect the actions of those who are stepping onto it. If I was successful the week prior to stepping on it, then the scale was my friend. If

I faltered and then tried to rationalize it, then the scale was a $%*&*#*@&* liar!

That's where my hatred for scales began. By stepping onto it, I was forced to address a part of me that I was not ready to deal with. But as I had embraced a life of truth, I found the scale to be a source of freedom rather than condemnation. I mean, realistically, if you never evaluate progress, you can never be held accountable for lack of success. I lived a life of destruction caused by ignorance and in all honesty, I was over excuses.

As autumn turned into winter and winter turned into spring:

1 Man
2 AA Batteries
3 Tapes in heavy Walkman rotation
4 Limbs working out to their limits
5 Bottles of water per day
6 a.m. every morning
7 Days a week
8 Months worth of blood, sweat, and tears
turned a broken shell of a boy into the amazing man you see before you. My transformation was so drastic that I even had the confidence to ask Mary Ann to my senior prom. She said yes. Jeremy Rochford, your life starts now!

Chapter 14:

It's Hard to Outrun Your Past When Your Shadow Is Larger Than You Are

...Or so it would seem. While our graduation slogan was "Every new beginning comes from some other beginning's end," I found myself struggling to find closure with most of the events in my past. Don't get me wrong, I was elated to finally tie my shoes the way they were designed to tie, laces in front instead of off to the side, but now it felt like people only spoke to me because of what I had accomplished. It seemed as though people were more interested in the story, than the person who created it. Girls who never acknowledged my existence or even the ones, who blamed the phantom farts on me, were inviting me to their graduation parties. The same guys who threatened me with violence merely because they could, asked me to go out and party with them. I imagine that is the same premise rappers feel when they talk about mo money, mo problems.

Success has an interesting way of changing people. It has the unique ability to draw them into vulnerable situations. I guess, for better or worse, I was not a person who could act like nothing happened. I had so many answers and explanations I felt owed to me before I could ever be social with any of those aforementioned people. Why did they never take the time to realize my weight was not the definition of my character? Why couldn't they realize it was an outward sign of dealing with issues the only way I knew how? Why did they take what little they thought they knew about me and use it to verbally abuse my existence for so long? Did they even realize that most of my emotional dysfunctions and the comfort I found in food were directly correlated from the social torment they put me through?

As everyone started to go their own way, I never thought I would ever get the vindication I deserved.

So?

What do you mean, so?

What do you mean, what do I mean?
Why in the world would you need someone else's
vindication after all you have accomplished?

I don't know. Because of all the
wrongs that needed to be made right?

I don' think that's the reason.

Oh really?
Then what is the reason?

To be honest, I think losing the weight has forced
"real Jeremy" to realize there is nothing holding him back.
I think you are clinging onto something from the past
so you won't have to face your fear of the future,
your fear of the unknown.

I never thought of it that way.

Honestly, I lived a life of not being good enough for so long, it was all I knew. Even with my success, I still had to shake off the hangover of that mentality. I never realized how mentally and emotionally abusive my relationship with food had become until I pulled myself out of it. It's hard to realize in the emotion of the moment, but the only one standing in my way of finding closure, was me.

As graduation gave way to summer work, summer work faded into my first year of college. Looking for a new start in every aspect of my life, I embraced every opportunity that higher education had to offer.

I made the effort to meet new people, experience new things, stay up way later than my parents ever would have allowed and even tried my best to wake up ridiculously early for class. While some efforts were more successful than others, the most purposeful experience was the effort I made to understand God's role in all of this.

Maybe it was the household I was brought up in, but I was always taught that if I were a good person and didn't do anything real crazy, then I would find God's favor and everything would work out in the end.

But if that was the case, then why did I have to experience such deep despair. My list of accomplishments read like a checklist for atonement. I was baptized at birth, an altar boy for years, went through catechism, confirmed, and regularly attended youth group all throughout high school. I even drove myself to church on Sunday mornings early enough to catch the pre-game bible study.

My discomfort for incompletes (and a few new friends),

lead me to seek a deeper understanding through some of the church sponsored bible studies on campus. I needed more of an explanation of God's greatness than habitual hand motions and camp songs. Unfortunately, that was all I got.

I think the pastor could see my frustration at points because he came over after the second meeting and asked me what I thought. I didn't want to insult him by saying that I didn't think my college experience would start like this, so I told him that he had a really nice guitar. Which he did.

Before I knew it, he placed the guitar in my hands and I was ripping through the only 4 chords I knew.

"Wow you play pretty well. You feel like leading worship sometime?" He said.

"Um no, not really" I replied.

"How come?" He asked.

"Argh...because I don't want to join your group." I thought to myself. I was hesitant to continue with any form of leadership because I knew that I wasn't going to school for ministry. But, I still said yes.

Honestly, I figured that I could use the friendship. Also, it was nice to have someone seek out my friendship instead of the other way around. However, as time progressed, I found that I developed a terrible habit of over-committing. I ended up binging on the attention. It was so new to me and I found that I wanted as much positive attention as I could get. In the long run, it set me up for a different kind of failure.

There was no efficient way to balance my involvement in leadership, academia, weekend employment, long-distance relationships, school life, home life, and well...any thing else.

I tried so hard to please everybody that in the end, I pleased nobody. My grades slowly faltered, my relationships became strained, work grew aggravated with me, my fellowship friends became slow to include me because I was still too "worldly," and my "worldly" friends became slow to include me because I was becoming too "Godly".

I had the hardest time trying to figure out exactly who I was. I felt like most of my identity was lost with all of my weight. In awkward situations, I used to just break the ice with a fat joke or something, but I no longer had that option. I was the last person able to carry on an educated conversation about anything other than why rollercoaster's lost their fun when they were executed safely and why ska music was surely a recurring fad.

Freshman year concluded, and I could firmly say my only success was my avoidance of the dreaded "freshman 15." Sophomore year began a little more hopeful, as I found myself in a relationship with someone who was seemingly as lost I was. We became acquaintances at first, and then it evolved into a legitimate friendship. I never pressed the issue for anything greater because I always assumed that ladies of her caliber (so smart, so pretty, so amazing in every sense of the word) would never have the patience to deal with someone who was as unsure of themselves as me. As it turned out, sometimes we're not always alone in being alone.

Charity and I were able connect in every sense of the word. By the time she accepted an internship that would take her 1000 miles away; I figured it was time for us to take a break.

Clearly not one of your prouder moments.

I know. I'm not saying it was.

I'm just sayin.

I know.

So why did you do it?
You could have just worked the
long distance relationship angle.

Yeah, but I was afraid and immature.
I don't know. I think that sometimes,
when you spend your entire life being told
 both verbally and non-verbally
that you are not good enough to be loved,
you start to believe it.
So when Charity and I became serious,
 I figured it would be easier to deal
with the loss of her 1000 miles away than
 it would be to have her come
back and watch it fall apart in front of me.

Aw, that's romantic.
Did you share that with her?

No

What? Why not?
What did you tell her?

That we should take a break
and see other people.

Are you serious? Really?
"We should take a break?"
That's the worst thing you could have told her.
What were you thinking?

Well, I guess I wasn't. Well, that's not true.
Since the day our eyes met I knew I was in love.
I just always figured I was on borrowed time.
Girls like her just don't end up with guys like me.
I figured that if we took a break now,
she would find someone who was better than me.
It was bound to happen anyway, and like I said, it's
a lot easier to deal with heartache
when it's 1000 miles away.

I see. So what happened?

Well, the short of it is that I went down
 to get her, and told her I loved her.
A year or so later, we got engaged,
 and then a year or so after that,
we got married.

Dude! Are you serious?
That's the perfect storybook ending.
Morbidly obese kid not only
goes on to lose the weight,
but he also gets the girl,
***and** lives happily ever after.*
You could not have written
a better ending to this story!

That's because I didn't.

What? Wait, what happened?

Well, first off, my freshman 15 arrived on a 12-month delay. While Charity was gone, I was so worried about losing her that I unconsciously went back to poor eating habits. I gained 15 pounds or so before I realized anything circumference wise had happened.

I didn't really think much of it because I had lost an additional ten in my first year, so to me, it all balanced out. Once she got back, we were so excited to just be around each other that fitness was the least of our concerns. My activities declined and another ten pounds crept on. Shortly after that, we were out of campus housing and into our own not-too-far-from-campus apartments. She would visit me at my place and I would have dinner at hers. She was such a great cook and it is hard to say no to a second plate of a home-cooked meal. That brought on another ten pounds. Soon, I quit hockey to focus on ministry. That brought on another 20-30 pounds.

Once I hit 270, I grew concerned. I began to go into a slight mode of panic. I entertained the idea of pills and even went for days without eating in hopes I would rekindle the once successful weight loss flame. I remember asking my housemate if he knew of any easy way I could lose a quick 20 pounds. He looked me dead in the eye and with a half-cocked smile he pointed to the gym and said, "The treadmill works every time."

I knew he was right. I had accomplished so much only two years prior. I knew exactly how this worked; the problem was that Charity and I became so comfortable with each other so quickly that staying in shape wasn't a priority for us. The next ten pounds went on with ease as I resolved myself to believe I needed caffeine and food to fuel my late night schoolwork and studies.

The final 30 pounds, well, I have no excuse for. The truth of the matter is that in a short three-year period, I went from celebrating the greatest victory of my life to looking as though nothing ever happened.

Chapter 15:

If We Are the Body, Then Why Are Our Thighs Rubbing?

I will never forget the day when God's still and quiet voice became so audible that I could no longer ignore it. While preparing an emo-tastical rendition of "In the Secret (I Want to Know You)" for our weekly fellowship, I somehow brought my acoustic guitar down at such an angle that the body of the guitar pinched my stomach between itself and my belt buckle. A little-known attribute of mine is my ability to unnecessarily over-rock acoustic songs which are clearly designed for pensive worship.

After feeling the warm sensation of bruising and almost instantaneous swelling, I quit playing to survey the damage. Putting the guitar down and lifting up my shirt, all of my focus was immediately drawn to the giant bruise that had amassed from all of the broken blood vessels and "rock" trauma. My first thought was, "Oh great, how am I going to explain this to Charity?" I mean, I knew that this mark was merely a bruise from an unnecessary guitar explosion...but I could see how a fiancée might easily mistake this for a hickey that was neither placed there by her, nor acceptable for our belief structure.

I put my head down and started to giggle at it. I figured our relationship endured the "let's see other people" fiasco, and she had personally endured multiple practice sessions where my worship theatrics were executed a little more accurately. I was confident she would understand exactly what happened.

As I raised my head from the carpet that facilitated all of this thought, my eyes caught the bruise one last time before they began to survey the rounded landscape surrounding it. I stared at my reflection for a moment. Reaching across my chest, I began to trace the fat creases and skin folds that had redeveloped. I looked up a little further and grabbed a piece of chest that for the past three years developed into a pectoral, but had now diminished back into moobage.

I turned 180 degrees to get a side perspective. My heart stopped beating. I could not believe how far over my pants I allowed my stomach to protrude. I looked down in hopes that at least I would still have visual contact with my feet. Instead of seeing a blue pair of skate shoes, all I could see was the pasty complexion of cellulite and failure. I dropped to my knees and began to cry. Why did I allow this to happen to me? Three short years ago my stomach was fully contained. Now, it's as though all of my hard work and triumph never even occurred.

Picking myself off of the floor, I kicked my guitar en route to the base of my bed. I stood there for a moment to catch my breath before I collapsed facedown into my comforter, which was in no way prepared for the amount of baggage it was about to receive. Without grace, my face sank in a myriad of blankets that nestled together to form a pillow-like mass upon my bed. Once landed, my heart sank even further. I cried harder. I cried so hard that I felt like my eyes would never recover. I had not cried for as long or as hard since the go-karting incident.

Once my tears dried up, time stood still for a moment. The weight of allowing every pound of the once lost weight to come back settled uncomfortably upon my shoulders. I felt sick and queasy. Then, the spiritual ramifications sunk in. I rolled over with all the conviction I could muster and began to speak at the ceiling. (The praying manifestation of God in my apartment was in the form of a mold-stained drop ceiling. I'm pretty sure it's not what he imagined on Calvary, but it worked for me). With a crackling voice I declared:

I can't do this any more God, I'm sorry.
After looking at myself in the mirror,
I just cannot lead worship in this condition.

I stared at the ceiling with the hopes of a divine reply. I knew that burning bushes were a little vintage, but my heart was dying for some form of communication from the suspended sheetrock. Receiving nothing but silence, I felt the need to explain myself further.

You see God, the thing is this...I love you,
and I know that ministry needs to occur.
The problem is, in this state, I'm not 100% sure
that I should be the one doing it. I mean,
doesn't it seem hypocritical for me to go
out suggesting there are more responsible ways for college students to handle their pre-marital relations as well as their perceptions of drug and alcohol use if I lack my own ability to responsibly handle an all-you-can-eat buffet? It just doesn't seem rational.
I'm not saying that I think food is sinful, I need to eat. But the problem I am having is that I keep running to food for all of the things **You're** supposed to be providing. I mean, how can I

honestly tell people that **You** are "More than enough", when I act like I don't believe it myself? I'm not sure what the solution is, but I feel pretty confident that it does not include me going out and misrepresenting you and Christianity to the masses.

I stared at the ceiling once more as I waited for God to speak to me with some form of vindicating comfort. What I heard was not what I expected.

You know Jeremy, while I agree that sometimes the church doesn't do an ideal job of reflecting my love for everyone accurately, it doesn't quite give you a reason to stop trying. If you authentically believe the Gospels encourage freedom and redemption, but there is something getting in the way of your life reflecting that, wouldn't it make sense to remove whatever part of your life is getting in the way?

Well, yeah, but I tried that once and here we are back again.

Eh...yes and no. James made a point in his scripture that faith without works is dead. It's a very solid principle. Think of that premise when you realize that emotion without direction will only lead to regress. Emotive situations provide short-term results because emotion, not solution, is propelling the effort. With no real solution, resolve and closure

are not found. That is why you gained
your weight back. You took the emotion of
eating and you angrily applied it to your weight loss.
Once the emotion of the situation had resolved
and the weight was lost, you never found a
healthy way to deal with how you felt about food.
There was just less of you, so when you
gained 5 or 10 pounds, it wasn't as noticeable.

So then, what is the answer?

Well, Jeremy, where you have been coming
up short in this weight loss struggle is that
you are trying to apply worldly solutions
to a God-sized problem. Food is not a sin by
any means. It never was and never will be.
How you approach food, well, we can talk about that later.
The bottom line is that in my first commandment
I stated that you should have no other God above me.
Not because I have a superiority complex,
I mean if I did, it would be justified, I am God after all.
But it is not for that reason. Being that I created you,
I know what is best for you. I see things that
you just can't see and more importantly,
I know that all of these other roads that draw you
away from me will only lead to failure.
Why do you think that every time you ran to
food for comfort, it was never enough?
Why do you think that every time you tried to
lose weight for vanity, it was never enough?
Why do you think that every time you ran
further away from me, I had to be more proactive

with getting your attention?
The school physical, the thyroid test, uncle Theo's cards.
Jeremy, every time you ran from what was best for you, what
you thought was punishment was
actually me trying harder to get your attention.
Jeremy, for far too long you did your best to
keep your God life and your real life separate.

Huh...?

You see, when you asked me to be the
Lord of your life, you never quite gave me the
room in your heart that I need to operate.
I was always sharing the space of your
heart with food. As the past few years transpired,
the space in your heart that you designated
for me became even less and less. When things
got troubling with Charity and school and so on,
instead of seeking first the kingdom
of God as the solution to your problems,
you sought comfort in eating.
If that is going to be your choice, then so be it.
That's the gift of free will.
But you can't invite me into your life with
the expectations of "Savior" and give me
little to no room to operate. If you want a more
casual relationship that's fine;
just don't be surprised
when we meet face to face and I say,
"I never REALLY knew you."
You just lost perspective that
some things have to change while
some things never should.

And while this burning bush moment was nothing more than an inner monologue between a stained drop ceiling tile and me, I knew unequivocally what God was trying to communicate to me.

It is the fundamental truth that I will never know peace in my life until I stop having a *spiritual* life, a *caloric* life, a *social* life, a *school* life, a *romantic* life, and I finally have just *one* life, with Jesus Christ overseeing all of it. When I finally took food out as lord of my life and gave Jesus the authority that He should have had all along, then and only then, was I able to find the closure I needed to walk (not run) away from my problems. More importantly, I was able to trade my fear of the perpetual failing moment for the faith in what I hoped tomorrow would bring.

I only had to believe in it.

That's where I find most of you right now. I can say these words because I was you, I am you. I have felt what you feel and I have feared what you fear. I also know that the same God who moved mountains in my life is the same God who can move mountains in yours. The only real question is, do you have enough faith to allow it to happen? That decision is yours and yours alone. Because of that, it no longer matters how *my* story ends, what matters most, is how **your** story begins.

This is your life...

Are you who you want to be?

More importantly...

Are you who Jesus wants you to be?

Acknowledgements

First and foremost I have to thank Jesus Christ. My hope is that this book reads less as a story and more of a testimony to what applied faith can accomplish. If faith can move mountains, this book shows what it can do for your waistline.

To my loving wife Charity, who has traveled and moved thousands of miles for us follow whatever our "calling" has been. Her guidance and patience has been the cornerstone that every successful person needs.

To my parents, whose support and encouragement never cease, no matter how embarrassing the truths of my past may be.

To Justin Lookadoo, this project would have never started if not for you. I am not sure there is a way to quantify your impact.

To Maverick and Media Design, your unwavering talent and support for this project can never be fully thanked.

To Mathew Paul Turner, the final inception of this book would not be nearly as cohesive if it wasn't for you.

To Geoff Hunker, Bob Morison, Allan Hardin, Sean Rogers, Brad Dunlap, Mike Harder, Courtney Furtner, Jeremy Willet, Nick Dewar, Mark Adkison, J.R. Mahon, Jai Brinkoski, Liam Slack, David Karkau, JB Brown, and Rich Furtner.

Finally, there have literally been hundreds of people who played some role in seeing this project come to fruition. There is no possible way to list everyone, but that does not diminish their impact. If you are one of those people, please place your name here:

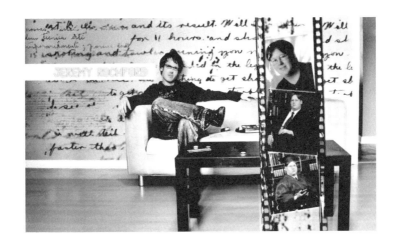

Jeremy Rochford is a weight loss success story, personal trainer, inspirational speaker, musician and all around nice guy. He lives in Nashville with his wife Charity and is always looking for his next challenge.

Currently, Jeremy is training for his first marathon where he hopes to raise money for underfed and malnourished children. For more information, social networking, live appreciates or personal training information, please visit:

JeremyRochford.com